AF520463

Clinical Guidelines for Management of Diabetes in Pregnancy

Federation of Obstetrics and Gynaecological Societies of India (FOGSI)

Clinical Guidelines for Management of Diabetes in Pregnancy

Editor-in-Chief

Pikee Saxena
MD (Obstetrics and Gynecology)
PGCC (Hospital Management) PGDCR
(Clinical Research) FICOG MNAMS FMAS
Professor
Department of Obstetrics and Gynecology
Lady Hardinge Medical College and
Smt Sucheta Kriplani Hospital
New Delhi, India

Editors

Alka Pandey
MD (Obstetrics and Gynecology) PhD FICOG FIMCH
Assistant professor
Department of Obstetrics and Gynecology
Patna Medical College and Hospital
Patna, Bihar, India

Anupam Prakash
MBBS MD (Gen. Medicine) PGCC (Hospital Management)
PDCDM FICP MAMS FACP FIACM
Professor
Department of Medicine
Lady Hardinge Medical College and
Smt Sucheta Kriplani Hospital
New Delhi, India

Forewords

Alka Kriplani MD FRCOG
FAMS FICOG FIMSA FICMCH FCLS

Yash Pal Munjal MBBS MD FICP MAMS FIAMS
FACP FIACMS FRCP (Edin)

JAYPEE *The Health Sciences Publisher*
New Delhi | London | Panama

Shalini Jaggi
Dip Diab (UK) Dip Endo (UK)
F Diab FRSSDI FRCP(Glasg Edin)
Consultant Diabetologist and Head
Dr Mohan's Diabetes Specialities Center
New Delhi, India

Sachin K Jain MBBS MD (Gen. Medicine)
FICP FACP FACE FRCP
Director Professor of Medicine
and Vice Principal
Lady Hardinge Medical College and
Associated Hospitals
New Delhi, India

Rita Kumari Jha MBBS MS PhD FICOG
Assistant Professor
Department of Obstetrics and
Gynecology
Patna Medical College and Hospital
Patna, Bihar, India

Rajesh Khadgawat MD (Medicine)
Professor, Department of Endocrinology
and Metabolism
All India Institute of Medical Sciences
New Delhi, India

Harsha Khullar
MD (Obstetrics and Gynecology)
Senior Consultant
Institute of Obstetrics and Gynaecology
Sir Ganga Ram Hospital
New Delhi, India

Anish Kumar
Research Associate
Internal Medicine
Max Super Speciality Hospital
Ghaziabad, Uttar Pradesh, India

Snigdha Kumari
MD (Obstetrics and Gynecology)
Assistant Professor
Department of Obstetrics
and Gynecology, ESI PGIMSR
New Delhi, India

Tarjani Makwana
MD (Ophthalmology)
Senior Resident
Dr Rajendra Prasad Centre for
Ophthalmic Sciences
All India Institute of Medical Sciences
New Delhi, India

Sonia Malik
MD (Obstetrics and Gynecology)
Program Director and
Head Southend IVF
New Delhi, India

Nihar Mehta MD (Medicine)
Joint Secretary
Associations of Physicians of India
Consultant Interventional Cardiologist
Jaslok Hospital and Research Center
KJ Somaiya Super Speciality Hospital
Bhatia Hospital
Mumbai, Maharashtra, India

Archana Mishra
MD (Obstetrics and Gynecology)
Associate Professor
Department of Obstetrics
and Gynecology
Vardhman Mahavir Medical
College and Safdarjung Hospital
New Delhi, India

Vandana Mohan MBBS
Resident
Department of Obstetrics
and Gynecology
Lady Hardinge Medical College and
Associated Smt Sucheta Kriplani Hospital
New Delhi, India

Sakshi Nayar
MS (Obstetrics and Gynecology)
Ex-Senior Resident
Department of Obstetrics and Gynecology
Lady Hardinge Medical College and
Smt Sucheta Kriplani Hospital
New Delhi, India

Aruna Nigam
MBBS MS FICOG MNAMS FMAS
Professor, Department of Obstetrics and Gynecology
Hamdard Institute of Medical Sciences and Research
Jamia Hamdard
New Delhi, India

Alka Pandey MD (Obstetrics and Gynecology) PhD FICOG FIMCH
Assistant Professor
Department of Obstetrics and Gynecology
Patna Medical College and Hospital
Patna, Bihar, India

Anupam Prakash
MBBS MD (Gen. Medicine) PGCC (Hospital Management) PDCDM FICP MNAMS FACP FIACM
Professor, Department of Medicine
Lady Hardinge Medical College and Smt Sucheta Kriplani Hospital
New Delhi, India

Bhanu Priya MD (Obstetrics and Gynecology)
Assistant Professor
Department of Obstetrics and Gynecology
University College of Medical Sciences and Guru Teg Bahadur Hospital
New Delhi, India

Manju Puri MD (Obstetrics and Gynecology)
Director Professor
Department of Obstetrics and Gynecology
Lady Hardinge Medical College and Associated Smt Sucheta Kriplani Hospital
New Delhi, India

Shalini Rajaram
MD (Obstetrics and Gynecology)
Director Professor, Department of Obstetrics and Gynecology
University College of Medical Sciences and Guru Teg Bahadur Hospital
New Delhi, India

Rekha Ramot
MSc (Nutrition and Dietetics), Registered Dietician
Department of Endocrinology and Metabolism
All India Institute of Medical Sciences
New Delhi, India

Asmita Muthal Rathore
MD (Obstetrics and Gynecology)
Director Professor
Department of Obstetrics and Gynecology
Maulana Azad Medical College
New Delhi, India

Tanushree Sahoo
MD (Padiatrics)
Senior Resident, Division of Neonatology
Department of Pediatrics
All India Institute of Medical Sciences
New Delhi, India

Pikee Saxena
MD (Obstetrics and Gynecology)
PGCC (Hospital Management) PGDCR (Clinical Research) FICOG MNAMS FMAS
Professor, Department of Obstetrics and Gynecology
Lady Hardinge Medical College and Smt Sucheta Kriplani Hospital
New Delhi, India

Gazala Shahanaz
MD (Obstetrics and Gynecology)
Fellowship of National Board of Examinations
High Risk Pregnancy and Perinatology
Maulana Azad Medical College and Hospital
New Delhi, India

Shalini MD (Obstetrics and Gynecology)
Resident
Patna Medical College and Hospital
Patna, Bihar, India

Siddharth N Shah MD (Medicine)
Hon Diabeteologist
Sir HN Reliance Hospital
Bhatia Hospital
SL Raheja Hospital
Saifee Hospital, Global Hospital
Mumbai, Maharashtra, India
Executive Editor— JAPI
Emeritus Editor—API Textbook of Medicine, Xth Edition

Ritu Sharma
MD (Obstetrics and Gynecology)
Associate Professor
Department of Obstetrics and Gynecology
NDMC Medical College and Hindu Rao Hospital
New Delhi, India

Abha Singh
MD (Obstetrics and Gynecology)
Director Professor and Head
Department of Obstetrics and Gynecology
Lady Hardinge Medical College and Smt Sucheta Kriplani Hospital
New Delhi, India

Narinder Pal Singh
MD (Medicine)
Medical Advisor and Senior Director
Internal Medicine
Max Super Speciality Hospital
Ghaziabad, Uttar Pradesh, India

Shweta Singh
MD (Obstetrics and Gynecology)
Senior Resident
Department of Obstetrics and Gynecology
ESI PGIMSR
New Delhi, India

Chitra Sinha
MD (Obstetrics and Gynecology)
Associate Professor
Department of Obstetrics and Gynecology
Patna Medical College and Hospital
Patna, Bihar, India

Raksha Soni
MD (Obstetrics and Gynecology)
Senior Resident
Department of Obstetrics and Gynecology
Lady Hardinge Medical College and Smt Sucheta Kriplani Hospital
New Delhi, India

Anshuman Srivastava
MD (Medicine)
Senior Resident
Department of Medicine
Lady Hardinge Medical College
New Delhi, India

Tanvi Tuteja MD
Consultant Obsterician and Gynecologist
Somaiya Super Speciality Hospital
Assistant Professor
KJ Somaiya Medical College and Hospital
Sunny Hospital
Chembur Apollo Spectra Hospital
Mumbai, Maharashtra, India

Pradeep Venkatesh
MD (Ophthalmology)
Professor
Dr Rajendra Prasad Centre for Ophthalmic Sciences
All India Institute of Medical Sciences
New Delhi, India

Foreword

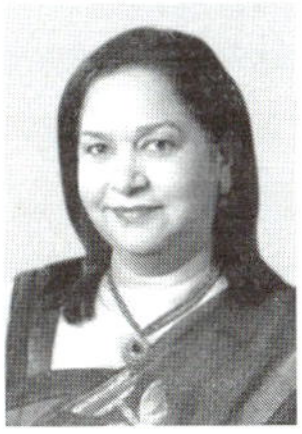

It gives me immense pleasure in congratulating Dr Pikee Saxena and her team for bringing out this book on *"Clinical Guidelines for Management of Diabetes in Pregnancy"*. Diabetes in pregnancy has become the new age epidemic which needs an awakening and awareness both among the physicians caring for the pregnant mothers and the endocrinologists who are involved at various stages. As they say, "Sugar is the new Tobacco" we can extrapolate it to saying "Diabetes is the new Menace". This book is a timely effort by Dr Pikee Saxena to bring to light the various aspects of this Disorder. There is an emphasis on beginning from basics of pathophysiology and maternal adaptations in diabetes to the pregnancy related issues like maternal and fetal afflictions. There are detailed sections on multi-pronged approach to management of Diabetes, from diet to oral hypoglycemics to Insulins.

This book will prove to be useful for obstetricians and endocrinologists alike.

Having worked with Dr Pikee Saxena in the past I know that she is a perfectionist and a stickler for detail and will ensure a high quality and standard for this project.

I wish all the very best to the Editors for this endeavour and hope that many practitioners and students will be benefited from this work.

Alka Kriplani MD FRCOG FAMS
FICOG FIMSA FICMCH FCLS
Professor and Head
Department of Obstetrics and Gynecology
All India Institute of Medical Sciences
New Delhi, India

Foreword

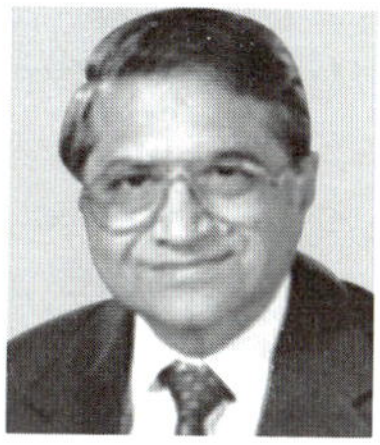

It gives me great pleasure to pen a Foreword for the book on *"Clinical Guidelines for Management of Diabetes in Pregnancy"*. Diabetes has assumed alarming proportions the world over and India is also grappling with the large numbers of diabetes individuals. Also, gestational diabetes has also increased over the last few decades. Therefore, diabetes and women in the reproductive age, are more related now. Also, the present theme of the International Diabetes Federation is "Women and Diabetes- our right to a healthy future". Therefore, this book is very pertinent, and is the need of the hour, importantly because there are not many texts on diabetes in pregnancy, though several texts exist on Gestational Diabetes. This happens to be a unique book since it comprehensively covers all the aspects of diabetes in pregnancy ranging from preconception to postpartum state including lactation period. This book also provides a peep in to the less commonly covered topics such as glycemic monitoring methods, bariatric surgery and also about the infant of a diabetic mother.

Moreover, this book presents an amalgamated view of both the Physicians and Endocrinologists on one hand and of the Obstetricians and Gynecologists on the other hand, which is seldom found in any single book. All the chapters in this book have been authored by senior faculty and practicing physicians/ gynecologists, and brings a whole lot of their expertise encapsulated in this book for the benefit of the readers.

The Editors of this book are renowned professionals, Dr (Professor) Pikee Saxena is a senior Faculty at the century old Lady Hardinge Medical College (LHMC), New Delhi, India and has several publications and original researches published. Dr Anupam Prakash, Professor of Medicine, LHMC is also a senior member of the Association of Physicians of India and is a renowned physician. Dr Alka Pandey is also a renowned obstetrician and gynecologist and a senior member of FOGSI.

I am sure that this book will provide for an illuminating reading for the readers, and will be well-received in the medical fraternity.

Yash Pal Munjal MBBS MD FICP MAMS FIAMS FACP FIACMS FRCP (Edin)
Director, Physicians' Research Foundation of
Association of Physicians of India (API), and Medical Director,
Banarsidas Chandiwala Institute of Medical Sciences, Okhla, New Delhi
Editor-in-Chief, API Textbook of Medicine-10th edition
Former President Association of Physicians of India
and Dean Indian College of Physicians

Preface

"Clinical Guidelines for Management of Diabetes in Pregnancy" is a comprehensive textbook containing vital information which is essential for the management of this common medical disorder. It aims to fill the gap in knowledge due to the lack of availability of management guidelines and provides important tips by experts from diverse specialities who are involved in the management of these patients. The book starts with **epidemiology of diabetes in pregnancy** in India and across the world. The chapters on **metabolic** and **pathophysiologic changes in diabetic pregnancy** will help the reader to understand the basis of various complications of hyperglycemia in pregnancy. Diabetes begets diabetes and the chapter on **intrauterine programming in diabetic pregnancy: future implications** discusses how hyperglycemia and other metabolic changes in diabetic pregnancy cause epigenetic changes and are responsible for intrauterine programming of the fetus which forms the basis on many adult onset diseases and intergenerational transmission of diabetes.

The chapter on **preconceptional counseling for women with diabetes** explains about the various precautions to be taken before conceiving in diabetic women to avoid maternal and fetal complications and have optimal pregnancy outcome. **Screening and Diagnosis of hyperglycemia in pregnancy** is a topic which is most controversial. There have been recommendations by different authorities, which have been changing many times over past several decades. An overview of the latest recommendations, their advantages and disadvantages, and the most practical screening strategy for our country including the National Guideline has been discussed in the chapter. There have been several advancements in methods used for measuring maternal plasma glucose. A separate chapter has been included on **glycemic goals and monitoring methods for Diabetes in pregnancy** including ambulatory and continuous glucose profile. Management of diabetes in pregnancy begins with **Medical nutrition therapy** including diet and **physical activity**. A chapter has been included for these important modalities. Patients who are not able to achieve glycemic control require pharmacotherapy including Insulin and oral antidiabetic therapy (OAD). Latest updates about **Insulin therapy in pregnancy: initiation, titration and safety** and current status of **OAD in pregnancy** will give a comprehensive knowledge about both. As diabetes in pregnancy is associated with high rate of stillbirths, a chapter is dedicated to **exploring causes of stillbirth in diabetic pregnancy** which has included new insight about the topic. Vascular complications like **diabetic nephropathy, diabetic retinopathy and hypertensive disorders in diabetic pregnancy** have been written by experts giving advice about their management during pregnancy. Chapters dedicated to **antenatal care and fetal monitoring in diabetic pregnancy, challenges in the management of macrosomia in diabetic pregnancy, intrapartum management, placenta in a diabetic pregnancy, managing the neonate of a diabetic mother** have been included in this book. Recognizing the importance of postpartum management in delaying or avoiding recurrent GDM, Type 2 diabetes a separate chapter covers all important aspects in the **postpartum/interconception management after gestational diabetes mellitus, breastfeeding** and **contraception in diabetic pregnancy**.

A chapter covers **perioperative management of pregnant women with diabetes** as they require special care during perioperative period. Obesity is becoming common all over the world and bariatric surgery is coming up as a new option for treatment of obese diabetic women. A chapter on **bariatric surgery: Impact on gestational diabetes** has been specially incorporated in the book. As many women with PCOS and type 2 diabetes suffer from infertility, abortions, a chapter on **fertility issues in women with hyperglycemia** also find a place in this text and make it a complete text on this subject. Controversial topics like continuation of Metformin and myoinositol during pregnancy have also been added.

The chapters include latest guidelines and management protocols, tables, flowcharts and key points which make it illustrative and very interesting for the readers. The book is intended to benefit the practicing clinicians and postgraduate students, and will enable them to manage diabetic pregnancies better, simultaneously improving obstetric and neonatal outcomes.

Pikee Saxena
Alka Pandey
Anupam Prakash

Acknowledgments

We wish to thank Dr Rishma Pai, President FOGSI and Dr Hrishikesh D Pai, Secretary General FOGSI for giving us the opportunity to write this book on *"Clinical Guidelines for Management of Diabetes in Pregnancy"* under the banner of FOGSI.

We deeply acknowledge our teachers and the patients who taught us and made us capable enough to gain knowledge and clinical experience to complete this book. We take this opportunity to thank our colleagues for their contributions and constant support for writing this book.

We are grateful to Ms Chetna Malhotra Vohra (Associate Director—Content Strategy) of Jaypee Brothers Publishers who was very active and cooperative in bringing out this book.

We wish to thank Dr Alka Kriplani, Immediate Past President, FOGSI and Head of the department of Obstetrics and Gynecology, AIIMS and Dr YP Munjal, Director, Physician's Research Foundation and Medical Director, Banarsidas Chandiwala Institute of Medical Sciences, Delhi for going through the book and writing the foreword.

We cannot thank our families enough for their unconditional support, encouragement and motivation that has made every achievement of ours possible and we wish to dedicate this book to them. We also thank the Almighty for His benevolence and never-ending blessings.

Contents

Plate-1

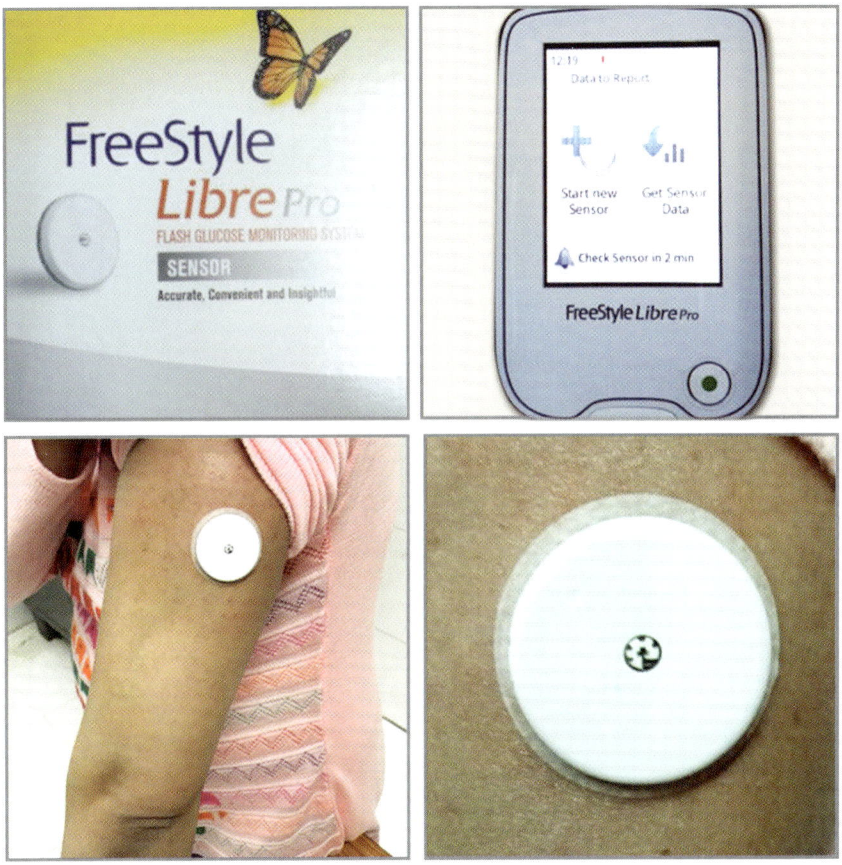

Fig. 1: Ambulatory glucose profile (AGP). Sensor device placed on a patient with a hand-held reader in the doctor's hand.

Plate-2

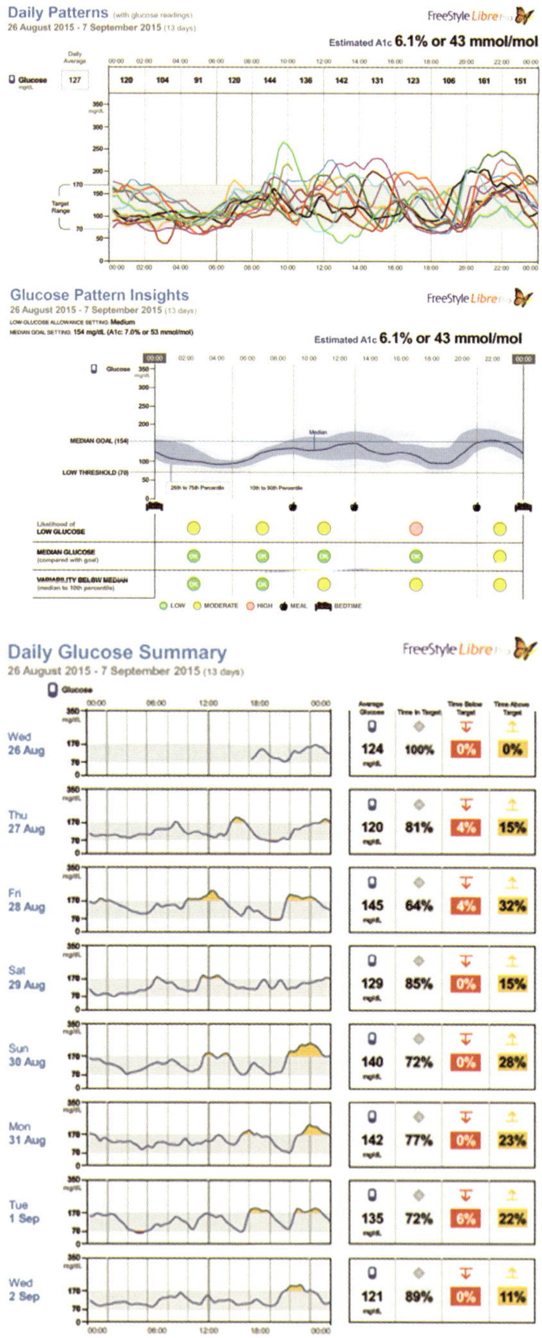

Fig. 2: Patterns obtained on 14 day Ambulatory Glucose Profile in addition to absolute values

Plate-3

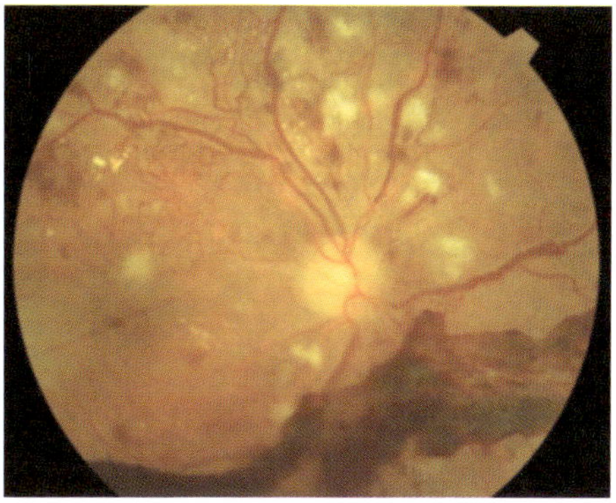

Fig. 3: Fundus photograph of the right eye of a patient with proliferative diabetic retinopathy. Neovascularization is noted along the superior arcade. Pre-retinal bleed is noted along the inferior arcade and inferior to the optic disk.

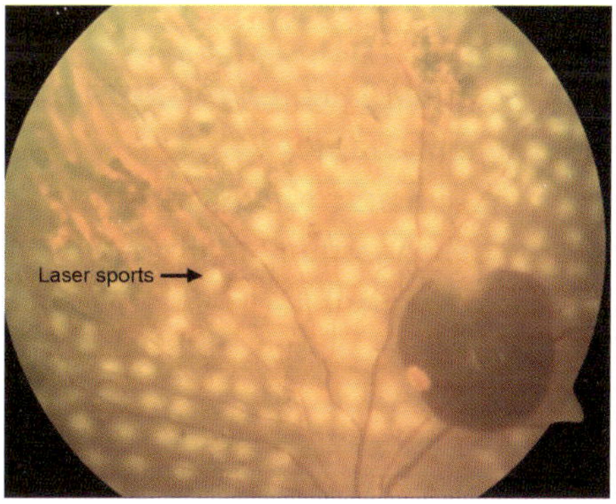

Fig. 4: Fundus photograph of a patient with proliferative diabetic retinopathy in which pan retinal photocoagulation has been performed. Fresh laser spots are seen (black arrow).

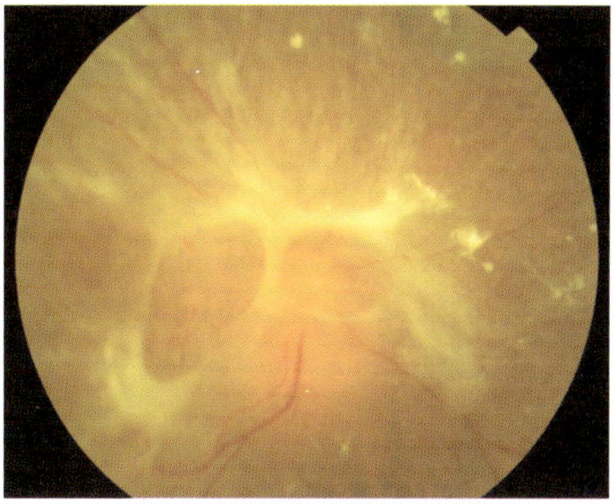

Fig. 5: Fundus image showing a large tractional retinal detachment extending from nasal to the optic disk toward the macula.

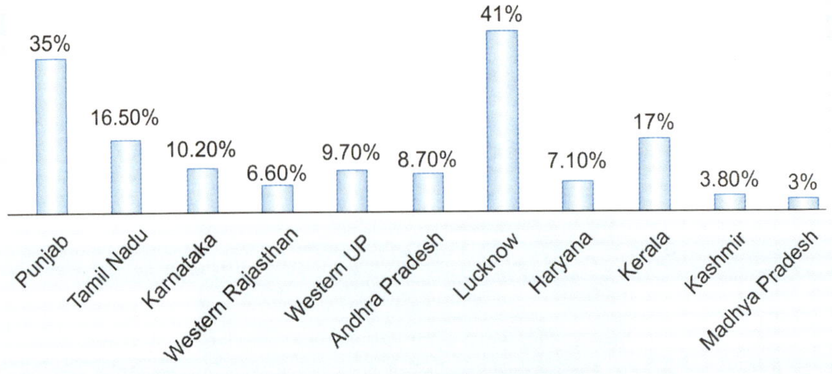

Fig. 1.1: Prevalence of gestational diabetes mellitus in different regions of India.

the prevalence of GDM in India was 2%,[8] which subsequently increased to 16.55% in 2000.[4]

The true prevalence of GDM remains variable due to variation in screening and diagnostic tests as well as due to ethnicity, which affects the prevalence rate without any bias.

Prevalence of GDM worldwide ranges from 1% to 14%;[9] while in India, it is between 3.8% and 21% in different regions of the country;[10] depending upon the geographical location, genetic makeup and method of diagnostic test used for screening.

Karnataka accounts for 10.2%, Tamil Nadu has 16.5%,[11] Andhra Pradesh has 12% and Kerala has 17%;[12] while central India like Madhya Pradesh has 3% rate and Kashmir has prevalence of 3.8%.[13] However, Haryana,[14] Uttar Pradesh[15] and western Rajasthan[16] have 7.1%, 9.7%, and 6.6% of prevalence according to the random studies. In more recent studies, using different criteria, prevalence rates as high as 35% from Punjab[17] and 41% from Lucknow have been reported (Fig. 1.1).[18] The geographical differences in prevalence have been attributed to differences in age and/or socioeconomic status of pregnant women in these regions. It is estimated that about 4 million women are affected by GDM in India, at any given time point.[19]

TREND

There is increasing trend of GDM nowadays due to changes in lifestyle, food habits, and reduced physical activity. Obesity has accelerated the onset of GDM in predisposed population. Earlier diabetes was considered as a disease of rich; but due to rapid urbanization, it is increasing in rural population also.

The prevalence of gestational diabetes is increasing globally and number of women with this condition is projected to rise from 171 million in 2000 to

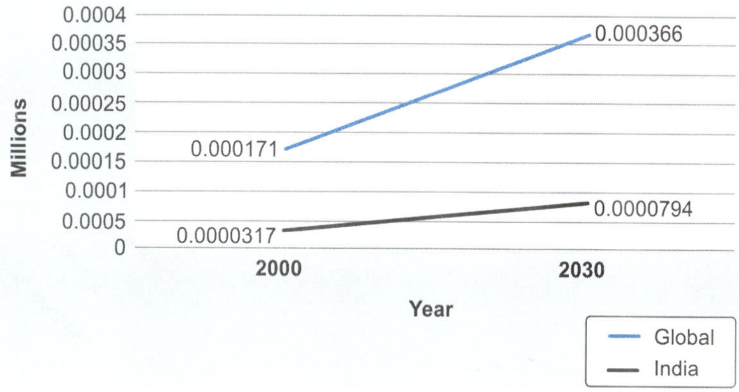

Fig. 1.2: Increasing prevalence of gestational diabetes mellitus (GDM).

366 million in 2030. India is expected to have 79.4 million in 2030 that will account for 15.1% increase from 31.7 million in 2000 (Fig. 1.2).[12]

Gestational diabetes mellitus contributes to about 90% of diabetes complicating pregnancy.[20] GDM imposes risks for both mother and fetus, some of which continues throughout the life of mother and child. Immediate maternal complications include preeclampsia, need for cesarean sections, and poly-/oligohydramnios.[21] Complications in the baby include hyperinsulinemia, macrosomia, shoulder dystocia, neonatal hypoglycemia, and respiratory distress syndrome. Women with GDM are at an increased risk of GDM in future pregnancies and also at a higher risk of developing Type 2 diabetes in the future.[22] GDM also increases the risk of obesity and glucose intolerance in the offspring.[23] GDM is therefore an important public health issue that has major repercussions for both mother and offspring. Detection of GDM thus provides a window of opportunity to intervene and reduce adverse perinatal outcomes.[24]

RISK FACTORS

There are various risk factors, which predispose a woman to develop GDM. Identification of those risk factors is important:

1. *Higher parity*
2. *Advanced maternal age*
3. *Family history of Type 2 DM:* Family history is significant because some genetic factors transmit from generation-to-generation among families. GDM in first-degree relative increases risk of GDM in patient. Managing diabetes is important not only to improve the maternal outcome but also avert diabetic risk across generations. Children born to diabetic

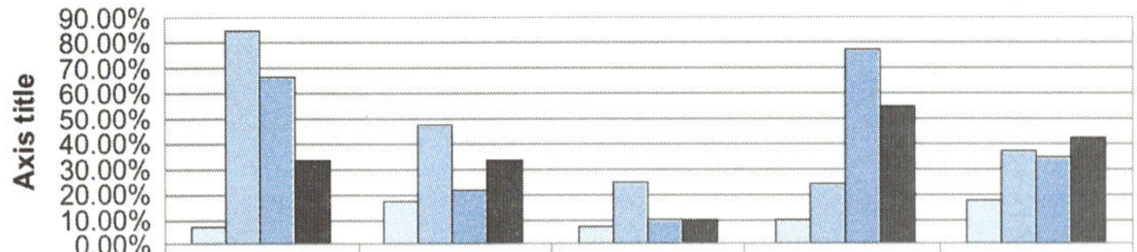

	Western Rajasthan 2013 (H)	Tamil Nadu 2005-2007 (E)	Haryana 2009-2011 (F)	Western UP 2014-2015 (F)	Kerala 2013-2014 (I)
Prevalence	6.60%	16.5%	7.10%	9.70%	17%
Age > 25 year	85%	47.30%	23.72%	22.70%	36.61%
BMI . 25 kg/m^2	66%	21.40%	8.24%	77.27%	33.33%
Family history	33%	32.30%	8.24%	54.54%	41.66%

Fig. 1.3: Comparison of various studies done in India. (BMI: Body mass index)

mother have impaired glucose intolerance and have metabolic complication; and in long-term, they have tendency to develop diabetes mellitus, obesity, and hypertension. Hence to decrease the prevalence of GDM, prevention of diabetes in mother is of paramount importance.

4. *History of big baby*: Due to lack of proper antenatal screening and lack of antenatal care (ANC) checkup, 60% of GDM is missed, but history suggestive of macrosomia in previous pregnancy raises the suspicion of GDM in present pregnancy.
5. *Caucasians/non-white race*: Due to genetic variation in different population, Caucasians have high-risk of genes for insulin resistance.
6. *History of perinatal loss*: Diabetes increases risk of sudden fetal demise, hence history of perinatal loss suggests that patient is high risk for developing GDM in this pregnancy.
7. *History of GDM*
8. *Obesity/overweight/body mass index (BMI) more than 25 kg/m^2*: Obesity accounts for 50% development of GDM. Lack of physical activity and exercise and also changes in diet eventually leads to obesity and hence increases risk of GDM. Routine ANC should include counseling regarding nutrition and physical activity, so that women gain appropriate weight during pregnancy.
9. *Lack of physical exercise and diet control*: Insulin resistance is main pathological key in developing GDM. Improving insulin sensitivity with exercise can decrease risk of diabetes (Fig. 1.3).

CONCLUSION

Diabetes hence is emerging as an epidemic in India. Due to lack of physical exercise, diet control and genetic predisposition of Indian population they are at risk to develop diabetes. Hence, health awareness, timely diagnosis, and lifestyle modification can decrease the morbidity associated with the disease.

KEY POINTS

- Diabetes is a major public health problem in India with prevalence rates reported to be between 4.6% and 14% in urban areas, and 1.7% and 13.2% in rural areas.
- Gestational diabetes mellitus contributes to about 90% of diabetes complicating pregnancy.
- Due to rapid urbanization , lack of exercise, poor diet habits it is increasing in rural population also.
- Detection of GDM provides a window of opportunity to intervene and reduce adverse perinatal outcomes.
- Postpartum followup of GDM is very important for early detection of Type II DM, hypertension and metabolic Syndrome.

REFERENCES

1. O'Sullivan JB. Gestational diabetes and its significance. In: Camerini-Davalos R, Cole HS (eds). Early Diabetes. New York: Academic Press; 1970:339-44.
2. American Diabetes Association. Gestational Diabetes Mellitus (Position Statement). Diabetes Care. 2004;27(Suppl 2):S88-90.
3. Schmidt MI, Ducan BB, Reichelt AJ, et al. For the Brazilian Gestational Diabetes Study Group. Gestational diabetes mellitus diagnosed with a 2-h 75 gm oral glucose tolerance test and adverse pregnancy outcomes. Diabetes Care. 2001;24:1151-5.
4. Seshiah V, Balaji V, Balaji MS, et al. Gestational diabetes mellitus in India. J Assoc Physicians India. 2004;52:707-11.
5. Anjana RM, Pradeepa R, Deepa M, et al. Prevalence of diabetes and prediabetes (impaired fasting glucose and/or impaired glucose tolerance) in urban and rural India: Phase I results of the Indian Council of Medical Research-INdia DIABetes (ICMR-INDIAB) study. Diabetologia. 2011;54:3022-7.
6. International Diabetes Federation. IDF Diabetes Atlas, 7th edition. Brussels, Belgium: International Diabetes Federation; 2015.
7. Dornhorst A, Paterson CM, Nicholls JS, et al. High prevalence of gestational diabetes in women from ethnic minority groups. Diabet Med. 1992;9:820-5.
8. Agarwal S, Gupta AN. Gestational diabetes. J Assoc Physicians India. 1982;30:203-5.
9. DeSisto CL, Kim SY, Sharma AJ. Prevalence Estimates of Gestational Diabetes Mellitus in the United States, Pregnancy Risk Assessment Monitoring System (PRAMS), 2007-2010. Prev Chronic Dis. 2014;11:130415.
10. Seshiah V, Balaji V, Balaji MS, et al. pregnancy and diabetes scenario around the world: India. Int J Gynaecol Obstet. 2009;104(Suppl 1):S35-8.
11. Seshiah V, Balaji V, Balaji MS, et al. Prevalence of Gestational Diabetes Mellitus in South India (Tamil Nadu)—A community Based Study. JAPI. 2008;56:329-33.
12. Sreekanthan K, Belicita A, Rajendran K, et al. Prevalence of Gestational Diabetes Mellitus in a Medical College in South India: A Pilot Study. Indian J Clin Pract. 2014;25(4):342-7.

13. Zargar AH, Sheikh MI, Bashir MI, et al. Prevalence of gestational diabetes mellitus in Kashmiri women from the Indian Subcontinent. Diabetes Res Clin Pract. 2004;66: 139-45.
14. Rajput FR, Yadav Y, Nanda S, et al. Prevalence of gestational diabetes mellitus & associated risk factors at a tertiary care hospital in Haryana. Indian J Med Res. 2013;137:728-33.
15. Swaroop GN, Rawat R, Lal P, et al. Gestational diabetes mellitus: study of prevalence using criteria of diabetes in pregnancy study group in India and its impact on maternal and fetal outcome in a rural tertiary institute. Int J Reprod Contracept Obstet Gynecol. 2015;4:1950-3.
16. Kalra HP, Kachhwaha CP, Singh HV. Prevalence of gestational diabetes mellitus and its outcome in western Rajasthan. Indian J Endocr Metab. 2013;17:677-80.
17. Arora GP, Thaman RG, Prasad RB, et al. Prevalence and risk factors of gestational diabetes in Punjab, North India: Results from a population screening program. Eur J Endocrinol. 2015;173:257-67.
18. Gopalakrishnan V, Singh R, Pradeep Y, et al. Evaluation of the prevalence of gestational diabetes mellitus in North Indians using the International Association of Diabetes and Pregnancy Study groups (IADPSG) criteria. J Postgrad Med. 2015;61:155-8.
19. Kayal A, Anjana RM, Mohan V. Gestational diabetes—An update from India, 2013. Diabetes Voice. 2013;58:1-5.
20. Expert Committee on the Diagnosis and Classification of Diabetes Mellitus. Report of the expert committee on the diagnosis and classification of diabetes mellitus. Diabetes Care. 2003;26(Suppl 1):S5-20.
21. Wendland EM, Torloni MR, Falavigna M, et al. Gestational diabetes and pregnancy outcomes—A systematic review of the World Health Organization (WHO) and the International Association of Diabetes in Pregnancy Study Groups (IADPSG) diagnostic criteria. BMC Pregnancy Childbirth. 2012;12:23.
22. Mpondo BC, Ernest A, Dee HE. Gestational diabetes mellitus: Challenges in diagnosis and management. J Diabetes Metab Disord. 2015;14:42.
23. Jovanovic L, Pettitt DJ. Gestational diabetes mellitus. JAMA. 2001;286:2516-8.
24. Mithal A, Bansal B, Kalra S. Gestational diabetes in India: Science and society. Indian J Endocrinol Metab. 2015;19:701-4.

CHAPTER 2

Metabolic Alterations in Diabetic Pregnancy

Siddharth N Shah, Nihar Mehta, Tanvi Tuteja

INTRODUCTION

Gestational diabetes is diabetes first detected in pregnancy. Although type 1 diabetes is more likely to develop in pregnancy, the great majority of women have pretype 2 diabetes, and many will go on to develop diabetes later in life. If type 1 diabetes is suspected during pregnancy or after delivery, autoimmunity should be confirmed by measurement of antibodies against islet cell antigens [antibodies directed against glutamic acid decarboxylase (GADA), islet antigen-2 antibody (IA-2A)]. Maturity onset diabetes of the young (MODY) may also present in pregnancy, and genetic testing is recommended when family history suggests that this phenotype may be present. However, in general gestational diabetes mellitus (GDM) can be regarded as pretype 2 diabetes.[1]

Gestational diabetes mellitus is a disease of the mother that associates with altered feto-placental vascular function. It describes a heterogeneous group of hyperglycemic metabolic disorders detected in pregnancy. It is characterized by inadequate beta cell secretion for the level of insulin resistance present whether the insulin response is normal or elevated.[2]

In normal pregnancy, insulin resistance emerges in the second trimester and progresses over the late third trimester, thereby increasing maternal glucose, free fatty acids (FFA), and amino acids in order to provide adequate energy to the fetus. In normal pregnancy, insulin resistance leads to an appropriate increase of insulin secretion, and blood glucose levels remain in the normal range. Due to the increasing demand of the developing fetus and increased transplacental nutrition transfer, maternal glucose levels are even lower than in healthy nonpregnant women.[1,3]

INSULIN RESISTANCE

The metabolic/endocrine changes accompanying the second half of gestation and inducing physiological pregnancy-related insulin resistance unmask and worsen the underlying pre-existing metabolic disturbances (pregestational insulin resistance and relative insulin secretion defect), leading to the full clinical picture of GDM.[4,5]

Impaired first phase insulin secretion, prolonged and increased second phase insulin release, reduced insulinogenic indices, increased hepatic glucose output (relative to prevailing hyperinsulinemia), changes in insulin kinetics, reduced glucose absorption from the gut, and varying degrees of insulin resistance have been described. These abnormalities have been described in women with GDM, as compared to pregnant women with normal glucose tolerance, based upon fasting or dynamic tests (oral and intravenous glucose tolerance tests).[1]

OTHER METABOLIC DISTURBANCES

Gestational diabetes mellitus associates with metabolic disturbances[1] such as abnormal handling of the locally released vasodilator adenosine, and biosynthesis and metabolism of cholesterol lipoproteins, or metabolic diseases resulting in endoplasmic reticulum stress and altered angiogenesis.

1. Increased fractional release of amylin and proinsulin relative to insulin secretion may be a cause or consequence of dysfunctional insulin secretion and action.[6] In addition, increased ectopic fat mass (intramyocellular and intrahepatic fat) and a slightly impaired flux through myocellular ATP synthase (fATP), the final step of mitochondrial oxidative phosphorylation, has also been found in women with GDM.[7]
2. Impaired lipid metabolism with increased FFA concentrations (insulin resistance of the adipose tissue with increased lipolysis) is also characteristic of the condition.
3. At present, changes of adiponectin and leptin appear to be the most important disturbances, although an increase of tumor necrosis factor-alpha (TNF-α) and plasma cortisol levels also parallel the increase of insulin resistance during pregnancy.[8]
4. TNF-α may impair the postreceptor insulin signaling cascade in skeletal muscle by activating pathways that increase sphingomyelinases and ceramides.
5. A decrease of adiponectin and increase of leptin has consistently been described, with changes in resistin, visfatin, chemerin, vaspin, fetuin-A, and many other proteins released from adipose tissue, the liver or the gastrointestinal tract have also been described, but with inconsistent results.[9]
6. Inflammatory markers such as C-reactive protein (CRP), interleukin-6 (IL-6), and soluble adhesion molecules [endothelial cell adhesion molecule (ECAM), vascular cell adhesion molecule (VCAM), and intercellular adhesion molecule (ICAM)] and vascular markers [e.g. asymmetric dimethylarginine (ADMA)] were found to be increased in some studies. In women with GDM or in those with a history of GDM, early endothelial dysfunction associates with the development of glucose dysregulation and other risk factors for atherosclerosis.

7. Another interesting association can be seen between bone markers and insulin secretion and sensitivity in GDM. Increased osteocalcin and C-telopeptide (CTX) levels in GDM could be regarded as compensatory mechanisms which try to cope with increased demand on insulin secretion, while decreased osteopontin levels may relate to insulin resistance in GDM.[10]

CONCLUSION

To conclude insulin is a key factor playing a modulatory role in GDM-associated altered angiogenesis, and metabolism of lipids in human fetoplacental vascular bed. Clinical management of insulin sensitivity is considered a therapeutic target in treatment of mothers with GDM and this could result in reversal of insulin resistance along with GDM-associated alterations in angiogenesis and lipid metabolism. Thus, a better understanding of the mechanisms behind the alterations along with treatment of these women with diet/exercise and insulin help in preventing adverse fetal outcomes from this disease.

REFERENCES

1. Pathogenesis of GDM. In: The Living Textbook of Diabetes. Available online at https://www.diapedia.org/41040851394/rev/19 Accessed on January 6, 2018.
2. Salzer L, Tenenbaum-Gavish K, Hod M. Best Pract Res Clin Obstet Gynaecol. 2015;29(3):328-38.
3. Kautzky-Willer A. Endocrine changes in diabetic pregnancy. In: Djelmis J, Desoye G, Ivanisevic M (Eds). Diabetology of pregnancy. Basel, New York: Karger; 2005. pp 18-33.
4. Xiang AH, Peters RK, Trigo E, et al. Multiple metabolic defects during late pregnancy in women at high risk for type 2 diabetes. Diabetes. 1999;48(4):848-85.
5. Catalano PM. Obesity, insulin resistance, and pregnancy outcome. Reproduction. 2010;140(3):365-71.
6. Kautzky-Willer A, Thomaseth K, Ludvik B, et al. Elevated islet amyloid pancreatic polypeptide and proinsulin in lean gestational diabetes. Diabetes. 1997;46(4):607-14.
7. Prikoszovich T, Winzer C, Schmid AI, et al. Body and liver fat mass rather than muscle mitochondrial function determine glucose metabolism in women with a history of gestational diabetes mellitus. Diabetes Care. 2011;34(2):430-6.
8. Buckley BS, Harreiter J, Damm P, et al. Gestational diabetes mellitus in Europe: prevalence, current screening practice and barriers to screening. A review. Diabet Med. 2012;29(7):844-54.
9. Worda C, Leipold H, Gruber C, et al. Decreased plasma adiponectin concentrations in women with gestational diabetes mellitus. Am J Obstet Gynecol. 2004;191(6): 2120-4.
10. Winhofer Y, Kiefer FW, Handisurya A, et al. CTX (crosslaps) rather than osteopontin is associated with disturbed glucose metabolism in gestational diabetes. PLoS One. 2012;7(7):e40947.

CHAPTER 3

Pathophysiologic Changes in Diabetic Pregnancy

Sandeep Garg, Jahnvi Dhar

INTRODUCTION

Diabetes mellitus (DM), commonly referred to as diabetes, is a group of metabolic disorders in which high blood sugar levels prevail over a prolonged period of time. It is due to either the pancreas not producing enough insulin or the cells of the body not responding properly to the insulin produced.

It is of three types:

1. *Type 1 DM:* Pancreas failure to produce enough insulin.
2. *Type 2 DM:* Begins with insulin resistance, a condition in which cells fail to respond to insulin properly. As the disease progresses a lack of insulin may also develop.
3. *Gestational diabetes:* Occurs in pregnancy without a previous history of diabetes.

Gestational diabetes is formally defined as any degree of glucose intolerance with onset or first recognition during pregnancy. This definition acknowledges the possibility that a woman may have previously undiagnosed DM, or may have developed diabetes coincidentally with pregnancy. Whether symptoms subside after pregnancy is also irrelevant to the diagnosis. A woman is diagnosed with gestational diabetes when glucose intolerance continues beyond 24–28 weeks of gestation.[1]

There are two subtypes:[2]

1. *Type A1:* Diet modification is sufficient to control glucose levels
2. *Type A2:* Additional therapy with insulin or other medications is required.

GDM encompasses various pathophysiological alterations which can have a profound impact on the pregnancy course with an adverse effect on the mother and the child. Various physiological alterations include:

- Hypertension (systolic and diastolic blood pressure)
- Dyslipidemia
- Thyroid dysfunction
- Insulin resistance (with/out metabolic syndrome)
- Increase in waist/hip ratio

- Hormonal imbalances (with their impact on future problems with diseases)
- Fetal outcome (with/out childhood obesity).

All these further can intermingle to generate risk for future systemic diseases in the mother and the child. Hence, they have to be dealt with aggressively with prompt institution of treatment.

HYPERTENSION

It is the most common medical problem encountered during pregnancy, complicating up to 10% of pregnancies.

Mechanisms for development of hypertension especially preeclampsia are:[3]

- Hyperglycemia stimulates vascular remodeling during implantation and placental development.
- Impairment of the cascade of vascular development predisposing to placental vascular compromise.
- Cytotrophoblasts organize placental remodeling during pregnancy, and excess glucose in diabetic pregnancy triggers intracellular changes in several stress signaling pathways resulting in cytotrophoblast cell dysfunction and abnormal placentation, thus development of preeclampsia.
- Insulin resistance may be a unifying factor in the occurrence of the two
- conditions together in pregnancy.

Hypertensive disorders during pregnancy are classified into four categories:[4]

1. *Chronic hypertension:* Defined as blood pressure exceeding 140/90 mm Hg before pregnancy or before 20 weeks gestation.
2. *Preeclampsia-eclampsia:* Preeclampsia is defines as gestational hypertension plus proteinuria (> 300 mg of protein in a 24-hour urine sample). Eclampsia is defined as the presence of tonic-clonic seizures appearing in a pregnant woman with high blood pressure and proteinuria.
3. *Preeclampsia superimposed on chronic hypertension.*
4. *Gestational hypertension (transient hypertension of pregnancy or chronic hypertension identified in the latter half of pregnancy):* Blood pressure higher than 140/90 mm Hg measured on two separate occasions, more than 6 hours apart, without the presence of protein in the urine and diagnosed after 20 weeks of gestation.

DYSLIPIDEMIA

There is an increase in total serum cholesterol and triglyceride (TG) levels in normal pregnancy and GDM, but these alterations are more profound in GDM with values increase by more than 15%.[5]

- The increase in TG levels is mainly as a result of increased synthesis by the liver and decreased lipoprotein lipase activity, resulting in decreased catabolism of adipose tissue.
- Low-density lipoprotein (LDL) cholesterol levels also increase and reach 50% at term. High-density lipoprotein levels increase in the first half of pregnancy and fall in the third trimester but concentrations are 15% higher than nonpregnant levels.[5]
- Changes in lipid metabolism accommodate the needs of the developing fetus. Increased TG levels provide for the mother's energy needs while glucose is spared for the fetus. The increase in LDL cholesterol is important for placental steroidogenesis.
- Rarer factors like subclinical inflammation, increased levels of apelin (adipocytokine), endothelial dysfunction etc. can also contribute.

THYROID DYSFUNCTION

There is an increase in the production of thyroxine-binding globulin (TBG) by the liver, resulting in increased levels of thyroxine (T_4) and triiodothyronine (T_3). Serum free T_4 (fT_4) and T_3 (fT_3) levels are slightly altered but are usually of no clinical significance. Levels of free T_3 and T_4 do however decrease slightly in the second and third trimesters of pregnancy and the normal ranges are reduced.[6] These changes are more profound in GDM which increases by more than 20.6% as compared to normal pregnancy.[6] All these changes have been suspected to be related to autoimmunity but no conclusive mechanism has been reported.

Serum concentrations of thyroid stimulating hormone (TSH) are decreased slightly in the first trimester in response to the thyrotropic effects of increased levels of human chorionic gonadotropin. Levels of TSH increase again at the end of the first trimester, and the upper limit in pregnancy is raised to 5.5 μmol/L compared with the level of 4.0 μmol/L in the nonpregnant state.[7]

INSULIN RESISTANCE WITH METABOLIC SYNDROME

GDM mothers are prone to have obesity, increased fasting insulin, high TG, and hypertension. Statistical differences were found on total cholesterol levels and fasting blood glucose (FBG) level between GDM and non-GDM mothers (both $P < 0.05$).[8]

- Placental derived hormones are believed to be a major factor in reprogramming maternal physiology to achieve an insulin-resistant state. However, with the exception of tumor necrosis factor alpha (TNF-α), changes in placental hormones in human pregnancy do not directly correlate with changes in maternal insulin resistance.[9]

- TNF may act in a paracrine fashion to contribute to skeletal muscle insulin resistance. TNF impairs insulin signaling by increasing serine phosphorylation of insulin receptor substrate (IRS)-1 and diminishing insulin receptor (IR) tyrosine kinase activity.[8,9]
- Dyslipidemia has shown to increase the risk of neural tube defects (NTDs) in GDM patients.

Metabolic syndrome is a clinical syndrome characterized as a complex of risk factors for cardiovascular diseases. Such patients may have DM, impaired glucose tolerance or insulin resistance complicated with hypertension, lipid disorders, atherosclerosis, proteinuria, and overweight or obesity. Thus, early prevention and immediate treatment is highly recommended for Metabolic syndrome.

INCREASE IN WAIST/HIP RATIO

Adipose tissue is preferentially deposited in the more metabolically active visceral compartment as pregnancy progresses. (visceral adipose tissue) VAT has an important role in metabolic and inflammatory responses, especially development of gestational hypertension and diabetes. Anthropometric measurements, such as waist circumference and waist-to-hip ratio, are often used as indirect measurements of visceral fat in nonpregnant adults.[10]

The increase in the waist/hip ratio is often used as a surrogate marker for the future risk of development of metabolic syndrome.

OTHER HORMONAL IMBALANCES

During pregnancy there is an increase in serum levels of deoxycorticosterone, corticosteroid-binding globulin (CBG), adrenocorticotropic hormone (ACTH), cortisol, and free cortisol. These changes cause a state of physiological hypercortisolism and may be clinically manifested by the striae, facial plethora, rising blood pressure, or impaired glucose tolerance. The hypothalamic-pituitary axis response to exogenous glucocorticoids is blunted during pregnancy. These changes occur in a similar magnitude in patients of GDM as compared to normal pregnancy, with no adverse effect to the fetus.[11]

The pituitary gland enlarges in pregnancy and this is mainly due to proliferation of prolactin-producing cells in the anterior lobe. Serum prolactin levels increase in the first trimester and are 10 times higher at term. The increase in prolactin is most likely due to increasing serum estradiol concentrations during pregnancy.[12] Levels of follicle-stimulating hormone (FSH) and luteinizing hormone (LH) are undetectable during pregnancy due to the negative feedback from elevated levels of estrogen, progesterone, and inhibin. Pituitary growth hormone production is decreased but serum growth hormone levels are increased due to growth hormone production from the placenta. These changes are not of a significant value in GDM patients.

The posterior pituitary produces oxytocin and arginine vasopressin (AVP). Oxytocin levels increase in pregnancy and peak at term. Levels of antidiuretic hormone (ADH) remain unchanged, but the decrease in sodium concentration in pregnancy causes a decrease in osmolality. There is therefore a resetting of osmoreceptors for ADH release and thirst.

PROTEIN METABOLISM

Pregnant women require an increased intake of protein during pregnancy. Amino acids are actively transported across the placenta to fulfill the needs of the developing fetus. During pregnancy, protein catabolism is decreased as fat stores are used to provide for energy metabolism. This especially holds true in GDM patients as they have an increased store of adipose tissue due to prevalent dyslipidemia.

CALCIUM METABOLISM

Increased calcium absorption is associated with an increase in calcium excretion in the urine and these changes begin from 12 weeks. During periods of fasting, urinary calcium values are low or normal, confirming that hypercalciuria is the consequence of increased absorption. Pregnancy is therefore a risk factor for kidney stones. These are not significant in GDM patients.

SKELETAL CHANGES WITH BONE LOSS

There is controversy regarding the effect of pregnancy on maternal bone loss. Although pregnancy and lactation are associated with reversible bone loss, studies do not support an association between parity and osteoporosis in later life. Bone turnover is low in the first trimester and increases in the third trimester when fetal calcium needs are increased. The source of the calcium in the third trimester is previously stored skeletal calcium.

Other musculoskeletal changes seen in pregnancy include:[13]

- Exaggerated lordosis of the lower back, forward flexion of the neck, and downward movement of the shoulders
- Joint laxity in the anterior and longitudinal ligaments of the lumbar spine
- Widening and increased mobility of the sacroiliac joints and pubic symphysis.

These changes have been reported in clinical trials to be more significant in patients of GDM as compared to normal pregnancy.

FETAL OUTCOME

It is well-acknowledged that the percentage of children with overweight or obesity is greatly increasing. More and more evidence proved that the health condition of mothers might contribute a lot to the development of obesity in the offspring.

In a study by Ameya R. Dudhwadkar[14] in 2016, maternal and fetal outcome in gestational DM was studied and following conclusions are mentioned below:

- Positive family history as a risk factor was noted in 20% patients.
- Polyhydramnios was found in 20%.
- 46% patients in this study delivered vaginally. 30% of vaginal deliveries were induced at 38 weeks of gestation while 70% went into spontaneous labor. 2% deliveries were vacuum assisted. 52% patients underwent lower segment cesarean section (LSCS).
- 78% of babies were born at term and 22% were preterm.
- Macrosomia and perinatal mortality are considered as adverse pregnancy outcomes in patients with GDM. 6% babies were intrauterine deaths. 40% babies were macrosomic at birth.
- Complications noted in neonates born to GDM mothers include fetal macrosomia, impaired fetal growth, metabolic and electrolyte abnormalities, cardiovascular and central nervous system (CNS) anomalies. 8% of the babies had hypoglycemia whereas 2% had hypocalcemia. In the present study, 8% had congenital anomalies.

CONCLUSION

Women with a history of GDM as well as offspring exposed to maternal diabetes in utero should be a major area of focus for preventive medicine. Preventive measures against type 2 DM should start during intrauterine period and continue throughout life from early childhood. Since, the only expenditure involved is a simple screening blood test; it is recommended that all patients be universally screened for GDM. In conclusion, a short-term intensive care gives a long-term pay off in the primary prevention of impaired glucose tolerance, diabetes and obesity in the offspring, as preventive medicine starts before birth.

KEY POINTS

- GDM encompasses various pathophysiological alterations which can have a profound impact on the pregnancy course.
- 10% pregnancies may be complicated by hypertension
- There is an increase in total serum cholesterol and triglyceride (TG) levels in normal pregnancy and GDM, but these alterations are more profound in GDM with values increased by more than 15%
- There is an increase in the production of thyroxine-binding globulin (TBG) by the liver, resulting in increased levels of thyroxine (T4) and triiodothyronine (T3).
- Placental derived hormones are believed to be a major factor in reprogramming maternal physiology to achieve an insulin-resistant state.

- Adipose tissue is preferentially deposited in the more metabolically active visceral compartment as pregnancy progresses. (visceral adipose tissue) VAT has an important role in metabolic and inflammatory responses, especially development of gestational hypertension and diabetes.
- During pregnancy there is an increase in serum levels of deoxycorticosterone, corticosteroid-binding globulin (CBG), adrenocorticotropic hormone(ACTH), cortisol, and free cortisol. These changes cause a state of physiological hypercortisolism and may be clinically manifested by the striae, facial plethora, rising blood pressure, or impaired glucose tolerance.
- Bone turnover is low in the first trimester and increases in the third trimester when fetal calcium needs are increased

REFERENCES

1. Mumtaz M. Gestational diabetes mellitus. Malays J Med Sci. 2000;7(1):4-9.
2. Gilmartin AB, Ural SH, Repke JT. Gestational diabetes mellitus. Rev Obstet Gynecol. 2008;1(3):129-34.
3. Brown CM, Garovic VD. Mechanisms and management of hypertension in pregnant women. Curr Hypertens Rep. 2011;13(5):338-46.
4. Anthony J, Damasceno A, Ojjii D. Hypertensive disorders of pregnancy: what the physician needs to know: review articles. Cardiovasc J Africa. 2016;27(2):104-10.
5. Pusukuru R, Shenoi AS, Kyada PK, et al. Evaluation of lipid profile in second and third trimester of pregnancy. J Clin Diagn Res. 2016;10(3):QC12-16.
6. Molehin D, Nitert MD, Richard K. Prenatal exposures to multiple thyroid hormone disruptors: effects on glucose and lipid metabolism. J Thyroid Res. 2016;2016:8765049.
7. Soma-Pillay P, Nelson-Piercy C, Tolppanen H, et al. Physiological changes in pregnancy: review articles. Cardiovas J Africa. 2016;27(2):89-94.
8. Zhang Y, Zhang HH, Lu JH, et al. Changes in serum adipocyte fatty acid-binding protein in women with gestational diabetes mellitus and normal pregnant women during mid-and late pregnancy. J Diabetes Investig. 2016;7(5):797-804.
9. Kirwan JP, Hauguel-De Mouzon S, Lepercq J, et al. TNF-α is a predictor of insulin resistance in human pregnancy. Diabetes. 2002;51(7):2207-13.
10. Berker D, Koparal S, Isik S, et al. Compatibility of different methods for the measurement of visceral fat in different body mass index strata. Diagn Interv Radiol. 2010;16 (2):99-105.
11. Lindsay JR, Nieman LK. The hypothalamic-pituitary-adrenal axis in pregnancy: challenges in disease detection and treatment. Endocr Rev. 2005;26(6):775-99.
12. Schock H, Zeleniuch-Jacquotte A, Lundin E, et al. Hormone concentrations throughout uncomplicated pregnancies: a longitudinal study. BMC Pregnancy Childbirth. 2016;16(1):146.
13. Ireland ML, Ott SM. The effects of pregnancy on the musculoskeletal system. Clin Orthop Relat Res. 2000;372:169-79.
14. Dudhwadkar AR, Fonseca MN. Maternal and fetal outcome in gestational diabetes mellitus. Int J Reprod Contracept Obstet Gynecol. 2016;5(10):3317-21.

CHAPTER 4

Intrauterine Programming in Diabetic Pregnancy—Future Implications

Rajesh Khadgawat, Rekha Ramot

INTRODUCTION

Diabetes during pregnancy could be result of one of the three reasons namely continuation of pre-existing type 1 or type 2 diabetes, or it may be new development of diabetes during pregnancy, which is often termed as gestational diabetes (GDM). In some cases, it may be continuation of secondary diabetes mellitus also, and occasionally maturity-onset diabetes of young (MODY) cases may be noticed. Diabetes in mother has been proposed to lead to an adverse intrauterine programming and unfavorable maternal environment causes inappropriate fetoplacental development and growth. Currently, the concept of intrauterine programming, although understanding is not very clear, refers to the ability of an adverse outcome during development to cause changes in physiology, metabolism, and epigenome of an individual and resultant increase in risk of chronic diseases at the long run. This concept includes changes at different developmental points and alterations resulting from a disturbance at the cellular, tissue, or organ level that can either be adaptive or in the intrauterine milieu, but will result in adverse outcome in postnatal period.[1]

PREVALENCE OF DIABETES IN PREGNANCY

Increased prevalence of diabetes during pregnancy has been noted in recent years, with much higher rise in GDM than type 2 and type1 diabetes. This rise in GDM parallels rise in type 2 diabetes in general population. In India, although it is difficult to predict any uniform prevalence across the country but results of published studies suggest a high prevalence of 10–15%. In a random survey performed in various cities in India, an overall GDM prevalence of 16.55% was observed. Another study from in Tamil Nadu showed 17.8% in urban, 13.8% in semiurban, and 9.9% prevalence of GDM in rural areas.[2] The rising prevalence of GDM reflects increasing prevalence of type 2 diabetes in general population from where all pregnant women are coming.

GLUCOSE METABOLISM IN NORMAL AND DIABETIC PREGNANCY

There are gradual changes in both basal and postprandial glucose metabolism during the course of pregnancy to meet the nutritional demands of the mother and fetus. These changes become evident as early as second trimester. During first trimester of pregnancy, basal glucose and insulin levels do not change much from nonpregnant state. However, as pregnancy progresses fasting blood glucose level decreases in spite of increase in endogenous hepatic glucose production. Increase in hepatic glucose production with a concomitant increase in fasting insulin is one of the important mechanisms. The other potential contributing factors behind these alterations include dilutional effects (increased plasma volume), increased utilization (either increased fetoplacental glucose utilization in late gestation or increased maternal uptake secondary to increased β-cell function). The summary of changes in maternal carbohydrate metabolism in normal pregnancy is listed below in the Table 4.1.

These adjustments take care of increased need of glucose by placenta and fetus. With advancement in pregnancy, insulin sensitivity also decreases, which may decrease up to 60–70% lower than normal nonpregnant subject. The physiologic factors responsible for decrease are partially related to the metabolic effects of several hormones and cytokines, which are elevated in the maternal circulation during pregnancy like human placental lactogen, progesterone, prolactin, and cortisol along with certain cytokines like TNF-α. This decrease in sensitivity is compensated by increase in secretion of insulin by maternal pancreas. By third trimester, insulin concentration may increase up to double of nonpregnant state. This increase in insulin secretion is contributed by both first and second phase of insulin secretion. Evidence from animal studies suggests an increase in β-cell mass resulting from a combination of β-cell hypertrophy and hyperplasia.[3]

Table 4.1: Changes in glucose metabolism during pregnancy compared to nonpregnant state.

Parameter	*Early pregnancy*	*Late pregnancy*
Basal metabolism:		
Fasting glucose	Unchanged	Decreased
Fasting insulin	Unchanged	Increased
Insulin metabolism		
Insulin secretion:		
First phase insulin secretion	Increased	Increased
Second phase insulin secretion	Increased	Increased
Insulin sensitivity	Decreased	Decreased

These changes in insulin sensitivity are more pronounced in obese pregnant women in comparison to nonobese pregnant women. Although the understanding of these changes is still not clear but changes in hormonal milieu during pregnancy is considered as one of the probable reasons.

IMPACT OF MATERNAL HYPERGLYCEMIA DURING PREGNANCY ON FETAL METABOLISM

As blood glucose moves freely across the placenta, hyperglycemia in mother is easily reflected on fetal circulation where increase in fetal blood glucose stimulates fetal pancreas to secrete more and more insulin to control this transferred high-blood glucose. Increased insulin, being an anabolic hormone, results in increase in size of cells and results in fetal macrosomia, one of the important complications of GDM if poorly controlled. Maternal hyperglycemia also results in increased uteroplacental glucose uptake with saturation kinetics that matches to the fetus without parallel rise in rate of uteroplacental oxygen consumption. Therefore, increased amount of glucose metabolized by placenta is shunted into nonoxidative pathways. Evidences from experimental animal studies have shown that chronic fetal hyperglycemia in response to maternal hyperglycemia results in downregulation of fetal pancreatic insulin secretion. As a result of the relative decrease in circulating insulin concentrations, fetal hyperglycemia is exaggerated, shifting the increased rate of uterine glucose uptake more into uteroplacental glucose consumption. Thus the uteroplacental glucose metabolism increasingly enters nonoxidative pathways.[4]

MECHANISM OF INCREASED RISK FOR CHRONIC DISEASE IN OFFSPRING OF DIABETIC MOTHER

The biological mechanisms explaining effect of maternal hyperglycemia during pregnancy on offspring's future health and diseases is still not well understood. There are data from animal studies suggesting that intrauterine exposure to hyperglycemia may induce disruptions in hypothalamic neurons, impairment of glucose metabolism, and β-cell dysfunction in pancreas in the offspring. These experimental findings are supported by data from epidemiologic studies suggesting that babies of diabetic mother are predisposed to fetal programming through increased insulin secretion, glucose intolerance, and altered inflammatory response. These changes in turn are found to be associated with childhood overweight/obesity and type 2 diabetes in adulthood.

Evidence for Perinatal Programming of Offspring of Diabetic Mothers

Data from animal studies on mechanisms whereby manipulation of fetal environment may result in adverse developmental programming of glucose intolerance and type 2 diabetes have been reported. A recently published review has suggested that the offspring of experimentally induced severe diabetic dams were small at birth and had decreased pancreatic weight and degranulated β-cells leading to low-pancreatic insulin content and low-plasma insulin. This resulted in insulin resistance in the offspring in the long run. However, in the same population, the offspring of mild diabetic rats had normal weight and enhanced percentage of pancreatic endocrine tissue, leading to higher β-cell mass and in long-term such offsprings have impaired glucose tolerance rather than insulin resistance.

Placenta of GDM mothers have shown characteristic histological changes such as villous immaturity, villous fibrinoid necrosis, chorangiosis, and increased angiogenesis. In early gestation, impaired glucose metabolism leads to structural dysfunctions; whereas in late gestation, placental function is affected causing inflammation and oxidative stress that can lead to the chronic fetal hypoxia. Short duration of diabetic insults in early gestation leads to limited fetal growth as a consequence of several placental adaptive responses including buffering excess maternal glucose or increased vascular resistance whereas longer duration of maternal hyperglycemia, hyperinsulinemia, or dyslipidemia will result in excessive fetal growth (macrosomia).

Available evidences from human studies suggest involvement of epigenetic mechanisms in the developmental programming of obesity and type 2 diabetes mellitus (T2DM) later in life. Studies from Pima Indian have supported the concept that intrauterine hyperglycemia modulates methylation of genes implicated in β-cell functions, thereby predisposing the offspring to increased risk of excessive adiposity and chronic lifestyle diseases later in life including diabetes. These studies provide an evidence of possible role of epigenetic mechanisms in contribution to long-term programming of obesity and metabolic disorders, but their authenticity is limited by small sample size, and also lack of independent replication; hence, the methylation changes detected often do not reach biological levels of significance.[5]

Long-term Consequences of Diabetes in Pregnancy on Offspring

Metabolic Syndrome and Obesity

Obesity is multifactorial in origin and results from complex interplay between genetic and environmental factors. Epidemiological longitudinal studies from Pima Indian population, a native homogenous tribal population with very high prevalence of type 2 diabetes have reported a link between hyperglycemia during pregnancy and development of obesity in offspring later on. It was reported that rates of obesity in children at ages 5–9, 10–14, and 15–19 years were higher in children born to women with diabetes during pregnancy in comparison to children born to mothers without diabetes during pregnancy. Even children born to mother with prediabetes also had higher body mass index (BMI) compared to children born to mother with normoglycemia. The mean BMI was 2.6 kg/m^2 higher in children who were exposed to hyperglycemia during pregnancy.[6] Another study from same population compared BMI between siblings who were born before development of GDM in mother and born during diabetes in pregnancy. It was found that children who were exposed to hyperglycemia during pregnancy had higher BMI in comparison to BMI of their siblings who were born before development of diabetes in mother hence were not exposed to hyperglycemia during pregnancy. Similar association of higher BMI at 1 year of age in children born to mothers with GDM in comparison to children born to mother with normoglycemia has also been reported in Caucasian population. In a recently published study, offspring of Caucasian women with GDM had a twofold increased risk of developing obesity and a fourfold increased risk of the metabolic syndrome compared to the background population.[7] This association has also been reported from multiethnic Enhanced Perioperative Care for High-risk Patients (EPOCH) study, where children of mothers with GDM had a higher increase in BMI and growth velocity than the unexposed controls, with the increase starting at the age of 10–13 years.

Type 2 Diabetes

Offspring of women with a history of diabetes during pregnancy are at increased long-term risk of developing insulin resistance and T2DM. The relation between birth weight and risk of T2DM is U-shaped and therefore both infants with lower and higher birth weight are at increased risk of developing T2DM as compared to persons being born with a normal birth weight. Studies from the Pima Indians have reported higher glucose levels during a 2-hour oral glucose tolerance test in early childhood (5–9 years of age) with higher prevalence of diabetes in 15–19-year-old children who were exposed to hyperglycemia during gestation in comparison to children did not. This prevalence of diabetes further increases from 20% at 15–19 years of age to approximately 50% by the age of 20–24 years of age. Children of diabetic mothers from Pima Indian population had been proposed to have a sixfold increased risk of developing T2DM compared to children born to nondiabetic mothers. Increased rates of impaired glucose tolerance has also been reported in children whose mother had diabetes from other populations.[8] Similar findings have also been reported in a study from Germany also where children born to diabetic mother had higher insulin, glucose and insulin glucose ratio at birth. These children also had higher prevalence of impaired glucose tolerance.

Cardiovascular and Renal Diseases

Offsprings of diabetic mothers have a worse cardiovascular risk profile, with increased levels of circulating cellular adhesion molecules, biomarkers of adverse endothelium perturbation, and compared with controls. Offspring of Pima mothers with diabetes during pregnancy also had higher systolic blood pressure than offspring of mothers who did not had diabetes, which persisted even after adjusting for adiposity.

Similarly, one study through in vitro and in vivo studies reported that exposure to a diabetic intrauterine environment to endothelial colony-forming cells (ECFCs) from newborns of diabetic pregnancies, reduced ECFCs colony formation and capillary-like tube formation and increased senescence and reduced proliferation. Therefore, infants born to diabetic mothers are predisposed to develop endothelial dysfunction and cardiovascular diseases (CVD) later in life. Angiotensin II (Ang II) can also be involved in the impairment of endothelial and vascular functions. An increase in cord blood Ang II concentration has been observed in offspring from mothers with GDM.[9]

Exposure to a diabetic intrauterine environment is also considered as a strong risk factor for renal disease. In Pima Indians studies, increased urinary albumin excretion (UAE) has been observed in the offspring of diabetic mothers (UAE was 58% in offspring of mothers with GDM, 43% in offspring of mothers who develop diabetes after pregnancy, and only 40% in offspring of nondiabetic mothers). These functional changes might result in damage to developing glomeruli possibly related to a similar process of nephron number decreased.[10] Among possible factors involved in the development of cardiometabolic diseases in offspring from diabetic mother, oxidative stress, and epigenetic alterations have been proposed.

Offspring Cognitive Impairment

Maternal diabetes during pregnancy has also been reported to have effect on fetal neurocognitive development and long-term cognitive ability. In a large Swedish record linkage study of 6,397 offspring of mothers with pregnancy diabetes and 1,300,683 children to mothers without diabetes, maternal diabetes during pregnancy was associated with a greater risk of not completing compulsory schooling at the age of 16 and with a lower mean school mark. Similarly, UK Avon Longitudinal Study of Parents and Children (ALSPAC), pre-existing diabetes, GDM and to a lesser extent, glycosuria were associated with lower offspring school entry assessment scores (at the age of 4 years), IQ (at 8 years), and school results (GCSE results, at 16 years), which persisted even after adjustment for potential confounders such as prepregnancy BMI, smoking during pregnancy, parity, mode of delivery, maternal education, and social class.[11]

In contrast to these two studies from population with relatively low rates of diabetes during pregnancy (0.5%), in Indian population with high prevalence of diabetes during pregnancy, offspring of women with GDM scored higher on a variety of cognitive tests compared with offspring of women without GDM at a mean age of 9.7 years, though after adjusting for a range of potential confounders, differences were somewhat attenuated toward the null.[6]

KEY POINTS

- Available evidence from human epidemiological studies, especially Pima Indian with high prevalence of diabetes has shown a possible association between role of exposure of fetus to intrauterine hyperglycemia and chronic diseases later in life.
- These studies report higher prevalence of obesity, metabolic syndrome, type 2 diabetes, hypertension, cognitive impairment, and renal diseases among children who were exposed to hyperglycemia during pregnancy in comparison to children who were not exposed.
- The exact pathogenesis of this increased risk is yet to be elucidated but a possible role of epigenetic changes have been proposed.

REFERENCES

1. Sutton EF, Gilmore LA, Dunger DB, et al. Developmental programming: state-of-the science and future directions-Summary from a Pennington Biomedical symposium. Obesity (Silver Spring). 2016;24(5):1018-26.
2. Rajput R, Yadav Y, Nanda S, et al. Prevalence of gestational diabetes mellitus & associated risk factors at a tertiary care hospital in Haryana. Indian J Med Res. 2013; 137:728-33.
3. Lain KY, Catalano PM. Catalano. Metabolic Changes in Pregnancy. Clin Obstet Gynecol. 2007;50:938-48.
4. Walker WA, Duggan C, Watkins JB. Text book of Nutrition in Pediatrics: Basic Science and Clinical Application, Volume 1, PMPH-USA, 2003. Hamilton: BC Decker; 2008. p 1102.
5. Monteiro LJ, Norman JE, Rice GE, et al. Fetal programming and gestational diabetes mellitus. Placenta. 2016;48:S54-S60.
6. Dabelea D, Pettitt DJ. Intrauterine diabetic environment confers risks for type 2 diabetes mellitus and obesity in the offspring, in addition to genetic susceptibility. J Pediatr Endocrinol Metabol. 2001;14:1085-91.
7. Clausen TD, Mathiesen ER, Hansen T, et al. Overweight and the Metabolic Syndrome in Adult Offspring of Women with Diet-Treated Gestational Diabetes Mellitus or Type 1 Diabetes. J Clin Endocrinol Metab. 2009;94:2464-70.
8. Pettitt DJ, Baird HR, Aleck KA, et al. Excessive obesity in offspring of Pima Indian women with diabetes during pregnancy. Diabetes Care. 1983;16:310-4.
9. Zhang F, Xiao X, Liu D, et al. Increased cord blood angiotensin II concentration is associated with decreased insulin sensitivity in the offspring of mothers with gestational diabetes mellitus. J Perinatol. 2013;33:9e14.
10. Atkins RC, Zimmet P. Diabetic kidney disease: act now or pay later. Acta Diabetol. 2010;47:1e4.
11. Fraser A, Nelson SM, Macdonald-Wallis C, et al. Associations of existing diabetes, gestational diabetes, and glycosuria with offspring IQ and educational attainment: the Avon Longitudinal Study of Parents and Children. Exp Diabetes Res. 2012;2012: 963735.

CHAPTER 5

Preconceptional Counseling for Women with Diabetes

Asmita Muthal Rathore, Gazala Shahanaz

INTRODUCTION

Diabetes is a state of glucose intolerance either due to insulin deficiency and/or insulin resistance. The American Diabetes Association (ADA) describes three classes of glucose intolerance in pregnancy—(1) type 1 diabetes, (2) type 2 diabetes, and (3) gestational diabetes mellitus (GDM).[1] Type 1 and type 2 diabetes exists before pregnancy and termed as pregestational diabetes. GDM term is used for glucose intolerance first diagnosed during pregnancy, but may include some undiagnosed pregestational diabetes. Also, there is a 7–9.6 times increased risk for developing type 2 diabetes later in life in cases of GDM.[2]

The incidence of diabetes among women of reproductive age and subsequently in pregnancy has been increasing over decades, largely because of shifts in dietary practices, reduced physical activity, and advanced age of conception. Majority (80–90%) are GDM and the rest type 1 and type 2 diabetes.[3]

Women suffering from chronic medical conditions including diabetes often have little knowledge about their disease status, pregnancy risks related to their condition, and how to optimize preconception health. The clinical practice guidelines of the American College of Obstetrics and Gynecologists (ACOG) and the ADA suggest that preconception care is an ideal primary prevention opportunity during which modifiable risk factors can be identified and reduced.

EFFECT OF DIABETES IN PREGNANCY

The knowledge of effects of diabetes in pregnancy is important for optimal preconceptional counseling. Normal pregnancy itself is a diabetogenic state associated with increased postprandial glucose levels and reduced insulin sensitivity due to the effects of various placental hormones, growth factors, and cytokines.[4] Maternal metabolic and vascular changes during pregnancy further affect glycemic control and increase the risk for progression of diabetes complications, which can contribute to poor pregnancy outcomes both maternal and neonatal. It includes spontaneous abortion, fetal anomalies, stillbirth, growth abnormalities, preterm delivery, birth trauma due to shoulder dystocia, as well as neonatal hypoglycemia and jaundice. Maternal complications for women with pregestational diabetes include worsening of pre-existing retinopathy and nephropathy, as well as increased risk for hypertension and preeclampsia.[3] It also increases the risk of obesity, type 2 diabetes, and cardiovascular disease in offspring later in life. The exact pathogenesis of these complications is believed to be multifactorial, but the risk of congenital malformations has been strongly associated with high-glucose concentrations during critical periods of development. Fetal hyperinsulinemia also contributes to neonatal morbidity.

In women with GDM, insulin resistance and hyperglycemia increase the risk for fetal macrosomia and birth complications.[1] In up to 30% of cases, GDM results in type 2 diabetes in mother 5–10 years postpartum[5] and obesity and metabolic syndrome in child.

PRECONCEPTIONAL COUNSELING

It is provision of multidisciplinary care before pregnancy, as fetal organogenesis is completed by 7 weeks of gestation, often before the woman knows she is pregnant. It includes an obstetrician, endocrinologist or physician, dietitian, and physical instructor for better management of glycemic control and diabetic complications. Women will undergo a full medication review—a review of diabetes-related complications, and an assessment for other conditions more commonly associated with diabetes and commence folic acid therapy.

Its main aim is to empower women with diabetes to have a positive experience of pregnancy and childbirth by providing information, advice, and support that will help to reduce the risks of adverse pregnancy outcomes for mother and baby.[6]

EFFECT OF PRECONCEPTION COUNSELING

Systematic reviews and meta-analysis supported an association between preconception care for diabetic women and improved glycemic control. The incidence of major congenital malformations can be reduced from 9% to 2% with preconception counseling.[7]

The effect of diabetes on health outcomes for mothers and their infants combined with observational evidence of the benefits of preconception care have prompted the implementation of preconceptual care for women with diabetes.[6]

The ADA recommended that all women with diabetes of childbearing potential should receive preconception counseling and that this counseling starts at puberty.

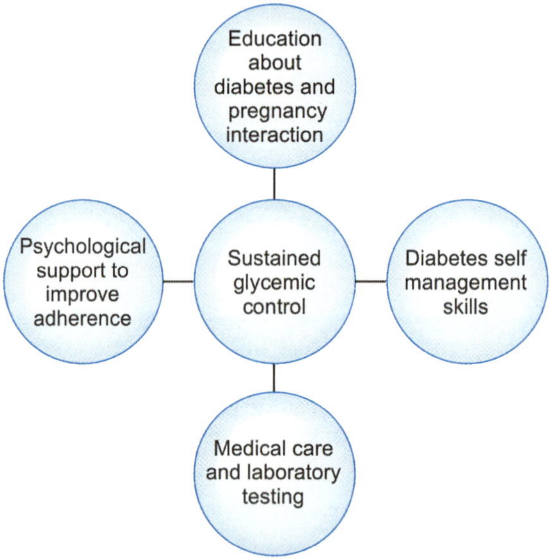

Fig. 5.1: Component of preconceptional counseling.

COMPONENT OF PRECONCEPTIONAL COUNSELING

It has four main elements:

1. Patient education about the interaction of diabetes, pregnancy, and family planning
2. Education in diabetes self-management skills
3. Physician-directed medical care and laboratory testing
4. Psychological support when indicated to reduce stress and improve adherence to the diabetes treatment plan (Fig. 5.1).

All elements are important to achieve the sustained glycemic control necessary to prevent congenital malformations and other complications.

Patient Education[1,6,8]

1. Information about effects of diabetes on pregnancy and how pregnancy affects diabetes.
2. Inform about role of diet, bodyweight, and exercise, the risks of hypoglycemia and impaired awareness of hypoglycemia during pregnancy, how nausea and vomiting in pregnancy can affect blood glucose control, the increased risk of having a baby who is large for gestational age and the likelihood of birth trauma due to shoulder dystocia, need for induction of labor and cesarean section.
3. Importance of near-normal glycemic (HbA1C—6.5%) before conception, if achievable without causing problematic hypoglycemia, as risk of diabetic embryopathy is directly proportional to elevations in A1C during the first 10 weeks of pregnancy.

4. Advise women that the risks increase with duration of diabetes and to use contraception until appropriate blood glucose control is achieved.
5. Emphasize the importance of avoiding an unplanned pregnancy as an essential component. Explain to women with diabetes that their choice of contraception should be based on their own preferences and any risk factors (if there are no standard contraindications to their use). All contraceptive methods are safe for women with history of GDM or pregestational diabetes unless they have vascular disease, nephropathy, retinopathy, neuropathy, or other comorbidities where estrogen-containing contraceptive methods should be avoided.
6. Explain about importance of maintaining good blood glucose control throughout pregnancy, which will further reduce the risk of miscarriage, stillbirth, and neonatal death. It is important to explain that risks can be reduced but not eliminated.
7. Explain the importance of good glycemic control during labor and birth and importance of early feeding of the baby to reduce the risk of neonatal hypoglycemia. Also explain the possibility of temporary health problems in the baby during the neonatal period, which may require admission to the neonatal unit and the risk of the obesity and/or diabetes in later life.
8. Inform them that extra-time and effort will be needed to manage diabetes during pregnancy and that she will have to frequently visit healthcare professional and make arrangements for support during pregnancy.
9. To start intake of folic acid (5 mg/day) before conception till 12 weeks of gestation to reduce the risk of having a baby with neural tube defect.
10. Encourage smoking cessation and reduction in alcohol intake.

Also screen for rubella, syphillis, hepatitis B, HIV, Pap smear, cervical cultures, and blood typing.

Diabetes Self-management Skills Education

1. Advise frequent monitoring of blood glucose including self-monitoring of plasma glucose and ketones before conception and monthly measurement of their HbA1c level.
2. Inform about plasma glucose targets and frequency of glucose monitoring.
3. *Target capillary plasma glucose*:
   - *Fasting*: 5–7 mmol/L on waking and
   - *Before meal*: 4–7 mmol/L at other time of the day
   - *After meals*: 5–9 mmol/L at least 90 minutes after eating.
4. Ensure individualized targets for self-monitoring of blood glucose with women who have diabetes and are planning to become pregnant, taking into account the risk of hypoglycemia.
5. Offer blood ketone testing strips and a glucometer, and advise them to test for ketonemia, if they become hyperglycemic or unwell.

6. Reassure women that any reduction in HbA1c level toward the target of 6.5% is likely to reduce the risk of congenital malformations in the baby.
7. Review medicines for treating diabetes including insulin and medicines for complications of diabetes.
8. Metformin may be used as an adjunct oral alternative to insulin in the preconception period, and during pregnancy, when the likely benefits from improved blood glucose control outweigh the potential risk for harm. All other oral hypoglycemic agents should be discontinued before pregnancy and insulin is substituted.
9. Isophane (NPH) insulin is the first choice for long-acting insulin during pregnancy. Long-acting insulin analogs (insulin detemir or insulin glargine) can be continued in women with diabetes, who have established good blood glucose control before pregnancy.
10. Data from clinical trials do not suggest that the rapid-acting insulin analogs (aspart and lispro) adversely affect the pregnancy or the health of the fetus or newborn baby.

Assessment of Complication and Associated Condition

1. An assessment of diabetes-related complications is commonly recommended as part of determining the progression of diabetes.[6]
2. A detailed history and examination to be done to assess duration and type of diabetes, presence of acute complications like infections, ketoacidosis, and hypoglycemia, and chronic complications, including retinopathy, nephropathy, hypertension, atherosclerotic vascular disease, and autonomic and peripheral neuropathy. This will provide information about how pregnancy may affect the progression of diabetes in the mother.
3. Offer retinal assessment at their first appointment and then annually, if no diabetic retinopathy is found.
4. Offer renal assessment, including a measure of albuminuria, before conception.
    - Referral to a nephrologist, if serum creatinine is above 120 μmol/L, the urinary albumin:creatinine ratio is greater than 30 mg/mmol or the estimated glomerular filtration rate (eGFR) is less than 45 ml/min/1.73 m^2, should be considered before discontinuing contraception.
    - Patients should be counseled about risks of hypertensive disorders of pregnancy and fetal growth restriction, if protein excretion is above 190 mg/24 hours or 400 mg/24 hours, respectively.[6]
5. Cardiovascular examination to be done for evidence of cardiac or peripheral vascular disease, and if found, patients should have screening tests for CAD before attempting pregnancy to assure they can tolerate the increased cardiac demands.
6. Consider neurological examination for signs of autonomic neuropathy.

7. Also look for associated medical conditions and medications, thyroid disease in particular for patients with type 1 diabetes, because of the 5–10% coincidence of hyper- or hypothyroidism.

Safety of Medicines for Complications of Diabetes before and during Pregnancy

1. Angiotensin-converting enzyme inhibitors and angiotensin-II receptor antagonists should be discontinued before conception or as soon as pregnancy is confirmed. Alternative antihypertensive agents suitable for use during pregnancy should be substituted.
2. Statins should be discontinued during periconceptional period.

Preconception Counseling in Women with Previous Pregnancy with GDM

Women with a normal glucose value in an index pregnancy have a minimal risk (<1%) that GDM will develop in a subsequent pregnancy within 4 years despite high-risk factors for gestational diabetes. GDM is more likely to recur in obese, parous women who had an early GDM diagnosis and required insulin in the index pregnancy. In addition, a shorter interval (≤24 months) and a larger weight gain (≥15 pounds) between pregnancies appear to be the most significant risk factors for a recurrence of GDM.[9]

Explain to women who were diagnosed with gestational diabetes about the risks of gestational diabetes in future pregnancies, and screen at 6–12 weeks postpartum using fasting plasma glucose (FPG) or 75-g, 2-hour OGTT, rescreen every 1–3 years.[10] GDM history should be discussed at all healthcare encounters. Pregnancy planning should include evaluation of glucose tolerance and, if abnormal, treatment of hyperglycemia before discontinuation of contraception. They should be offered early self-monitoring of blood glucose or an OGTT in future pregnancies. A subsequent OGTT should be offered, if the test results in early pregnancy are normal.

It is concluded that the control of weight gain and interval between pregnancies could be important to reduce GDM recurrence. Subsequent diabetes risk after a history of GDM is significantly lower in women who followed healthy eating patterns.

This concurs with the recommendation that preconceptional counseling in gestational diabetics is required to improve glucose homeostasis before conception and throughout pregnancy, and that appropriate evaluation of glucose intolerance should be included as part of prospective family planning.

BARRIERS TO PRECONCEPTIONAL CARE[11]

- Gaps in knowledge of clinician and women with diabetes
- Limited resources and time.

- Difficulty in targeting patients who are planning conception.
- High prevalence of unintended pregnancies (50%), representing missed opportunities to maximize a woman's health status before conception.[12]
- Poor attention to recommended screenings is another barrier. Despite recommendations to screen for type 2 diabetes after pregnancy, the postpartum screening rate for women with GDM is only ~50%,[13] representing a missed opportunity to enhance wellness before future pregnancy occurs.

IMPROVING UPTAKE OF PRECONCEPTION CARE

- Explain to women with diabetes about the benefits of preconception blood glucose control at each contact with healthcare from adolescence.
- Document the intentions of women with diabetes regarding pregnancy and contraceptive use at each contact with their diabetes care team from adolescence.
- Ensure supportive environment, and encourage the woman's partner or other family member to attend counseling.

KEY POINTS

- Use a multidisciplinary preconception care team.
- Perform a full medical and obstetric evaluation in the preconception period to assess risks.
- Evaluate and treat diabetic complications before pregnancy, including retinopathy, nephropathy, neuropathy, and cardiovascular disease including hypertension.
- Measure and optimize thyroid hormone levels in women with type 1 diabetes.
- Review all current medications, and change to a form of therapy that has less fetal risk.
- Assess level of metabolic control. Measure HbA1C monthly until control is achieved. HbA1C should remain below 6.5%, if possible.
- Manage blood glucose levels to achieve optimal pregnancy glycemic goals preconceptionally without hypoglycemia. Educate on hypoglycemia awareness and management.
- Selection of antihyperglycemic therapy. Insulin should be prescribed for type 1 and type 2 diabetic patients, because the safety of currently available oral antidiabetic agents is not assured during early pregnancy.
- Commence folate supplementation, 4 mg daily from before conception until 12 weeks' gestation to minimize congenital anomalies.
- Provide information about risks of miscarriage, congenital malformation, and perinatal mortality with poor metabolic control and unplanned pregnancy. Inform about how DM affects pregnancy and how pregnancy affects DM.

- Use effective contraception until target blood glucose control is achieved before conception.

REFERENCES

1. American Diabetes Association. Management of diabetes in pregnancy. Sec 12. In Standards of Medical Care in Diabetes—2016. Diabetes Care. 2016;39(Suppl.1):S94-8.
2. Bellamy L, Casas JP, Hingorani AD, et al. Type 2 diabetes after gestational diabetes: a systematic review and meta-analysis. Lancet. 2009;373:1773-9.
3. American College of Obstetricians and Gynecologists. (2017). Pregestational diabetes mellitus. [online] Available from http://www.acog.org/-/ media/Practice-Bulletins/ Committee-on- Practice Bulletins Obstetrics/pb060. [Accessed December, 2017].
4. Vargas R, Repke JT, Ural SH. Type 1 diabetes mellitus and pregnancy. Rev Obstet Gynecol. 2010;3:92-100.
5. Shaat MN, Almgren P, Groop L, et al. Prediction of postpartum diabetes in women with gestational diabetes mellitus. Diabetologia. 2010;53:452-7.
6. NICE guideline. (2015). Diabetes in pregnancy: management from preconception to the postnatal period. [online] Available from nice.org.uk/guidance/ng3. [Accessed December, 2017].
7. American Diabetes Association. Standards of medical care in diabetes—2009. Diabetes Care. 2009;31(Suppl 1):S40-1.
8. American College of Obstetricians and Gynecologists. (2005). The importance of preconception care in the continuum of women's health care (Committee Opinion No. 313). [online] Available from http://www.acog.org/-/media/Committee-Opinions/ Committee-on-Gynecologic Practice/co313.pdf?dmc=1&ts=20150829T1739406986. [Accessed December, 2017].
9. Kim C, Berger DK, Chamany S. Recurrence of gestational diabetes: a systematic review. Diabetes Care. 2007;30:1314-93.
10. Metzger BE, Buchanan TA, Coustan DR, et al. Summary and recommendations of the Fifth International Workshop-Conference on Gestational Diabetes Mellitus. Diabetes Care. 2007;30(Suppl 2):S251-60.
11. Dunlop AL, Jack B, Frey K. National recommendations for preconception care: the essential role of the family physician. J Am Board Fam Med. 2007;20:81-4.
12. Finer LB, Zolna MR. Unintended pregnancy in the United States, 2001-2008. Am J Public Health. 2014;104(Suppl 1):S43-8.
13. Tovar A, Chasan-Taber L, Eggleston E, et al. Postpartum screening for diabetes among women with a history of gestational diabetes mellitus. Prev Chronic Dis. 2011;8:A124. [online] Available from http://www.cdc.gov/pcd/issues/2011/nov/11_0031.htm. [Accessed December, 2017].

CHAPTER 6

Screening and Diagnosis of Hyperglycemia in Pregnancy: Challenges and Controversies

Pikee Saxena, Aruna Nigam

INTRODUCTION

Pregnancy is a diabetogenic state due to a number of hormones such as placental lactogen, growth hormone, and corticotropin-releasing hormone, secreted primarily by the placenta. Traditionally, gestational diabetes mellitus (GDM) is defined as onset or first recognition of abnormal glucose tolerance during pregnancy.[1] The American College of Obstetricians and Gynecologists (ACOG) still uses this terminology.[2] The disadvantage of this terminology is that it fails to differentiate between the women who develop insulin resistance during pregnancy from those who already have preexisting diabetes. Different terminologies have been used to classify hyperglycemia during pregnancy. Recently, the International Federation of Gynecology and Obstetrics (FIGO) has attempted to recognize those women who already have preexisting diabetes. Hence, the following terms have been coined:[3]

- *Gestational diabetes mellitus:* Diabetes recognized in second half of pregnancy or not meeting the criteria for overt or pregestational diabetes.
- *Diabetes in pregnancy:* Hyperglycemia detected before the start of pregnancy or diagnosed for the first time during pregnancy meeting the criteria for overt or pregestational diabetes. It may be type 1 or type 2. The world prevalence of GDM is 6–7.7%[4] and in India it is 16.5%.[5]

SIGNIFICANCE OF SCREENING

Diabetes in pregnancy is associated with several adverse outcomes for the mother and the fetus (Table 6.1). The Hyperglycemia and Adverse Pregnancy Outcome (HAPO) study demonstrates that maternal hyperglycemia, even at a level below the diagnostic threshold of diabetes, is associated with increased birth weight and macrosomia.[6] It has been observed that the adverse outcomes increase as the maternal plasma glucose level increases in a continuous manner.[6,7]

Besides the above mentioned maternal, fetal, and neonatal complications, the offspring of a GDM mother is exposed to hyperglycemia in the

Table 6.1: Pregnancy complications associated with hyperglycemia in pregnancy.

Maternal	*Fetal and Neonatal*
Spontaneous miscarriage	Congenital malformations
Preeclampsia	Macrosomia
Polyhydramnios	Fetal growth restriction
Infections	Increased operative injuries
Operative delivery	Intrauterine death
Postpartum hemorrhage	Neonatal hypoglycemia
End organ damage	Neonatal hyperbilirubinemia
Cardiovascular disease	Neonatal respiratory distress

intrauterine period which causes epigenetic changes[8] resulting in childhood obesity, impaired glucose tolerance (IGT), hypertension, and type 2 diabetes mellitus later in life. Therefore, it is important to screen and diagnose hyperglycemia early in pregnancy and initiate treatment to prevent pregnancy complications for both the mother and fetus, and also to avoid intrauterine programming of the fetus to avert fetal origin of adult disease.

Whom to Screen?

There are two schools of thought:

1. *High risk or selective screening:* ACOG[2] and National Institute for Health and Care Excellence (NICE, 2015)[9] recommend screening for hyperglycemia only in high-risk populations
   I. Risk factors:
      A. Body mass index (BMI) >30 kg/m^2
      B. Previous macrosomic baby weighing > 4.5 kg
      C. Previous still birth or anomalous baby
      D. Previous history of gestational diabetes
      E. Family history of diabetes (first-degree relative)
      F. High-risk ethnic population for diabetes mellitus—African, Asians, and non- Caucasians
      G. History of polycystic ovarian syndrome (PCOS)
2. *Universal screening:* Screening of the entire population or sub group irrespective of the risk factors is recommended by American Diabetes Association (ADA),[10] International Association of Diabetes and Pregnancy Study Group (IADPSG)[6] and Diabetes in Pregnancy Study Group India (DIPSI).[5]

In a previous study, risk-based screening for GDM recognized 1.45% of women as against universal screening which recognized 2.7% in the same population showing that risk-based screening had missed half of the cases of GDM.[11] In India, universal screening is needed, as Indian women have 11-folds increased risk of developing glucose intolerance in pregnancy as compared to Caucasian women.[5]

When to Screen?

Data from human and animal studies have correlated the existence of chronic diseases such as obesity, diabetes mellitus, and cardiovascular diseases to the perinatal nutrition due to a process known as early metabolic imprinting.[8] Hence, screening should be done in the first trimester to identify those women who already have preexisting diabetes. Early detection and initiation of treatment helps to control the sugar levels and avoids complications in the mother and the offspring by modifying the nutrition at an early gestation. Different international authorities recommend screening at different gestations as shown below:

- NICE: 24–28 weeks in high-risk population[9]
- ACOG: 24–28 weeks, except, women with high-risk factors who are screened at first visit[2]
- ADA and IADPSG: First antenatal care (ANC) visit and then at 24–32 weeks in previously undiagnosed GDM[10,6]
- DIPSI: First visit, if normal then at 24–28 weeks and repeat at 30–32 weeks.[5]

How to Screen and Diagnose?

A universal guideline for the ideal screening and diagnosis method is lacking. A number of methods have been suggested on the basis of population risks, cost-effectiveness, and lack of large national screening programs.

ACOG

ACOG 2017[2] continues to recommend two step procedure:

1. Step 1: Glucose challenge test (GCT)/glucose loading test (GLT)
   I. 50 g oral glucose load irrespective of last meal
   II. If 1 hour venous plasma glucose >140 mg/dL, proceed to second step
   III. If 1 hour venous plasma glucose ≥200 mg/dL, then a diagnosis of pregestational diabetes is made
2. Step 2: Glucose tolerance test (GTT)
   I. After an overnight fast of 8–10 hours and 3 days of unrestricted diet, measure fasting plasma glucose
   II. Give 100 g of glucose load
   III. Blood is then drawn at hourly intervals (three samples).

ACOG recognizes both Carpenter-Coustan and National Diabetes Data Group (NDDG) criteria[12] to diagnose GDM. Table 6.2 depicts thresholds for plasma glucose values for diagnosis of GDM in pregnancy.

Table 6.2: ACOG thresholds of plasma glucose values for diagnosis of gestational diabetes mellitus.

Time	*Carpenter-Coustan*[2,11]	*NDDG*
Fasting	95 mg/dL	105 mg/dL
1 hour	180 mg/dL	190 mg/dL
2 hours	155 mg/dL	165 mg/dL
3 hour	140 mg/dL	145 mg/dL

(ACOG: American College of Obstetricians and Gynecologists; NDDG: National Diabetes Data Group).

If any two or more of the mentioned values are deranged, the condition is labeled as GDM. The limitations of ACOG criteria is that cutoffs are not based on fetal or maternal morbidity. Cutoffs identified those women who are at high-risk of developing diabetes after pregnancy. For this test, two visits are required and five blood samples are drawn which causes inconvenience to the women, is time consuming and costly.

NICE

The NICE 2015[10] recommends that if women have high-risk factors, 75 g oral glucose tolerance test (OGTT) should be done as soon as possible. If it is negative, test should be repeated again at 24–28 weeks. Women without any risk factors should be screened at 24–28 weeks. For screening, 2-hour 75 g OGTT is done in a fasting state. Thresholds of plasma glucose values for diagnosis of GDM are given below in Table 6.3.

Table 6.3: NICE thresholds of plasma glucose values for diagnosis of gestational diabetes mellitus.

Time	*Plasma glucose (mg/dL)*
Fasting	≥100
2 hour	≥140

(NICE: National Institute for Health and Care Excellence)

IADPSG

The IADPSG criterion[4,5] has been adopted by ADA in 2010 and by World Health Organization (WHO) in 2013. Based on the HAPO study, cut-off levels for diagnosis of GDM were lowered to give an odd's ratio of 1.75 times the likelihood of adverse outcomes (fetal birth weight, cord C peptide, and percent body weight >90% percentile) at mean glucose levels of HAPO study.[6,7] They observed that adverse pregnancy outcomes, like fetal macrosomia, preeclampsia, primary cesarean delivery, neonatal adiposity, and cord blood

Flowchart 6.1: IADPSG criteria for diagnosis of hyperglycemia in pregnancy.

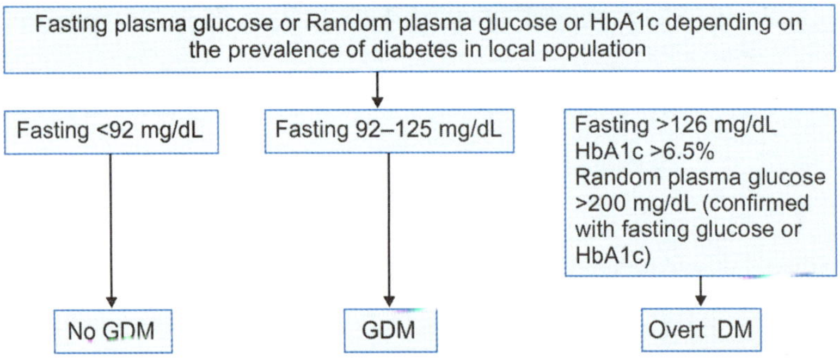

(IADPSG: International Association of Diabetes and Pregnancy Study Group; HbA1c: hemoglobin A1c; DM: Diabetes mellitus; GDM: Gestational diabetes mellitus)

Table 6.4: IADPSG threshold of plasma glucose for diagnosis of gestational diabetes mellitus.

Time	*Plasma glucose(mg/dL)*
Fasting	≥92
1 hour	≥180
2 hours	≥153

(IADPSG: International Association of Diabetes and Pregnancy Study Group)

C-peptide levels were noted even below the threshold of diagnostic criteria of GDM (< 95 mg/dL).

The IADPSG recommends screening during first trimester by fasting or random plasma glucose or hemoglobin A1c (HbA1c) (Flowchart 6.1) and if negative a repeat one step, diagnostic, 2-hour 75 g OGTT is done at 24–28 weeks. Plasma glucose is determined at 0 hour, 1 hour, and 2 hours, and if any one value is above threshold, woman is labeled as GDM (Table 6.4).

If fasting plasma glucose is more than or equal to 126 mg/dL or any value i.e. random, postprandial, or postglucose is more than or equal to 200 mg/dL, overt or pregestational diabetes is diagnosed. This is the only criterion for diagnosing GDM which is based on risk of adverse pregnancy outcome. Although, IADPSG criteria has been recommended by WHO and ADA, it is time consuming, costly, and inconvenient as three blood samples need to be drawn and the patient has to come in a fasting state for a second visit.

ACOG stated that lowering the thresholds of diagnosis of GDM in IADPSG would result in increasing the prevalence and hence, the cost of health care.[2]

Seshiah et al.[5] debated that IADPSG had the following limitations:

- The Asians have higher insulin resistance in pregnancy and hence increased blood glucose levels, unlike Caucasians on whom HAPO study was conducted

- Mostly, pregnant women do not come fasting to the hospital and if asked to come back in a fasting state, the dropout rate is very high, especially in developing countries.

ADA

ADA 2017[10] recommends either one step IADPSG criteria or two step ACOG criteria mentioned above for screening and diagnosis of GDM.

DIPSI

Keeping in mind the high prevalence of diabetes in India and considering the low ANC coverage and lack of infrastructure, diabetes in pregnancy study group, India have suggested a universal, one step screening and diagnostic procedure (Table 6.5).[5] Blood sugar is estimated 2 hours after 75 g of oral glucose load given to the pregnant woman at the first ANC visit, irrespective of the last meal.

Table 6.5: Interpretation of DIPSI for diagnosis of hyperglycemia in pregnancy.

Plasma glucose level (mg/dL)	*Diagnosis*
≥140–199	Gestational diabetes mellitus
≥200	Pregestational diabetes

(DIPSI: Diabetes in Pregnancy Study Group India)

We evaluated the efficacy of DIPSI with WHO GTT in a tertiary care hospital of Delhi. It was observed that out of the 800 pregnant women evaluated, 51 were diagnosed as GDM by WHO criteria, 63 by DIPSI. The sensitivity of DIPSI test with respect to WHO 1999 was 98.04% and specificity 98.26%. The diagnostic accuracy of DIPSI was 98.25% and the area under the receiver operating characteristic curve (ROC) for DIPSI was 0.988 ($p < 0.001$) (95% confidence interval: 0.960–1.000).[13] The scientific validity of DIPSI has also been proven by several other studies.[14,15] However, another study reported sensitivity of DIPSI test for diagnosis of GDM to be low.[16]

DIPSI is a one step, simple, convenient, and economical test for diagnosis of GDM. Only a single blood sample needs to be drawn. As DIPSI test is done in the nonfasting state, it reduces the chances of missing the diagnosis of GDM in a pregnant woman who may not come back in a fasting state during the next visit. Due to these advantages, DIPSI criteria has also been recommended by the Ministry of Health and Family Welfare for diagnosis of GDM in India.[5]

WHO

WHO 1999[17] states that hyperglycemia first detected at any time during pregnancy should be classified as either diabetes mellitus in pregnancy or GDM.

Table 6.6: Interpretation of WHO 1999 OGTT for diagnosis of hyperglycemia in pregnancy.

Plasma glucose level (mg/dL)	*Diagnosis in pregnancy*	*Diagnosis outside pregnancy*
≥140–199 after 75 g glucose load	Gestational diabetes mellitus	Impaired glucose tolerance
>126 fasting	Pregestational diabetes	Diabetes mellitus
≥200 random or after 75 g glucose load	Pregestational diabetes	Diabetes mellitus

(WHO: World Health Organization; OGTT: Oral glucose tolerance test)

Plasma glucose is measured in a fasting state and then 2 hours later after a 75 g OGTT. Pregnant women who meet the criteria for IGT are classified as having GDM (Table 6.6).

WHO used the same interpretive criteria for pregnant women as that for nonpregnant women. It is not based on fetal or maternal complications associated with hyperglycemia and this criterion is based on the risk of developing diabetes mellitus. As it is a simple one step test involving only two blood samples, it became popular in many countries.

As the fasting plasma glucose of 126 mg/dL was considered to be quite high, a need was felt to update the WHO 1999 criteria. Therefore, WHO in 2013 adopted the IADPSG criteria for diagnosing diabetes in pregnancy.[18]

CONCLUSION

As Indians belong to high-risk ethnic group with high prevalence of diabetes, early universal screening for diabetes is recommended at the first antenatal visit. The IADPSG criteria is the only outcome based criteria, it has the ability to diagnose and treat GDM earlier, thereby reducing the fetal and maternal complications associated with GDM. This one step method is accurate and is close to international consensus but it is inconvenient, costly, and increases the prevalence of GDM due to lower thresholds.

Therefore, in low resources and rural areas where it is not feasible to carry out the IADPSG diagnostic test, DIPSI is recommended as a sensitive, one step, convenient, and economical diagnostic test with least disturbance to patient's routine activities (Table 6.7).

KEY POINTS

- Diabetes in pregnancy has been associated with serious adverse effects on the mother and fetus. It has been seen that an early detection and management helps to avoid these harmful effects. Hence, the need for universal screening and early diagnosis is of paramount significance.

Table 6.7: Summary of all screening tests for diagnosis of hyperglycemia in pregnancy.

Organization	*Year*	*Screening mode*	*Approach*	*Glucose load*	*Diagnostic criteria (mg/dL)* Fasting	1 hr	2 hr	3 hr	*Remarks: Diagnosis of GDM*
ACOG	2013	Universal	Two step	100 g	95	180	155	140	Carpenter and Coustan; ≥2 value abnormal
					105	190	165	145	NDDG; ≥2 value abnormal
NICE	2015	Selective	One step	75 g	100	-	140	-	≥1 value abnormal
WHO	2013	Universal	One step	75 g	92	180	153	-	≥1 value abnormal
ADA and IADPSG	2010	Universal	One step	75 g	92	180	153	-	≥1 value abnormal
DIPSI	2006	Universal	One step	75 g	-	-	140	-	1 value

(ACOG: American College of Obstetricians and Gynecologists; NICE: National Institute for Health and Care Excellence; WHO: World Health Organization; ADA: American Diabetes Association; IADPSG: International Association of Diabetes and Pregnancy Study Group; DIPSI: Diabetes in Pregnancy Study Group India; NDDG: National Diabetes Data Group)

- There is a lack of uniform consensus on the methods of screening and diagnosis of diabetes in pregnancy.
- Clinician should understand the evidence but individualize decision making according to the specific patient or situation.
- For low- and middle-income countries with high-diabetic burden, universal, early screening with single step, DIPSI criteria appears to be convenient and evidence based.
- In India, DIPSI criteria is advocated by the Ministry of Health and Family Welfare for diagnosis of GDM.
- IADPSG criteria which has been adopted by WHO and ADA may be followed when feasible.

REFERENCES

1. Proceedings of the 4th International Workshop-conference on Gestational Diabetes Mellitus. Chicago, Illinois, USA. 14-16 March 1997. Diabetes Care. 1998;21 Suppl 2:B1- 167.
2. Committee on Practice Bulletins—Obstetrics. Practice Bulletin No. 180: Gestational Diabetes Mellitus. Obstet Gynecol. 2017;130(1):e17-37.
3. Hod M, Kapur A, Sacks DA, et al. The International Federation of Gynecology and Obstetrics (FIGO) Initiative on gestational diabetes mellitus: A pragmatic guide for diagnosis, management and care. Int J Gynaecol Obstet. 2015;131 Suppl 3:S173.
4. Shaw JE, Sicree RA, Zimmet PZ. Global estimates of the prevalence of diabetes for 2010 and 2030. Diabetes Res Clin Pract. 2010;87(1):4-14.
5. Seshiah V, Sahay BK, Das AK, et al. Diagnosis and Management of Gestational Diabetes mellitus: Indian guidelines. Diabetology. 2013;44(5):201-04.
6. Metzger BE, Gabbe SG, Perrson B et al. International association of diabetes and pregnancy study group recommendations on the diagnosis and classification of hyperglycemia in pregnancy. Diabetes Care. 2010;33(3):676-82.
7. Metzger BE, Lowe LP, Dyer AR, et al. Hyperglycemia and adverse pregnancy outcomes. N Eng J Med. 2008;358(19):1991-2002.
8. Waterland Robert A, Garza Cutberto. Potential mechanisms of metabolic imprinting that lead to chronic disease. Am J Clin Nutr. 1999;69(2):179-97.
9. NICE. (2015). Diabetes in pregnancy: management of diabetes and its complications from preconception to postnatal period. NICE guidelines. [online] Available from http://www.nice.org.uk/guidance/ng3/evidence [Accessed December 2017].
10. American Diabetes Association. Classification and Diagnosis of Diabetes. Diabetes Care. 2017;40 (Suppl 1):S11-24.
11. Griffin ME, Coffey M, Johnson H, et al. Universal versus risk factor based screening for gestational diabetes mellitus detection rates, gestation at diagnosis and outcome. Diabet Med. 2000;17:26-32.
12. O'Sullivan JB, Mahan CM. Criteria for oral glucose tolerance test in pregnancy. Diabetes. 1964;13:278-85.
13. Saxena P, Verma P, Goswami B. Comparison of Diagnostic Accuracy of Non-fasting DIPSI and HbA1c with Fasting WHO Criteria for Diagnosis of Gestational Diabetes Mellitus. J Obstet Gynecol India. 2017. 67(5):337-42.
14. Sharma K, Wahi P, Gupta A, et al. Single glucose challenge test procedure for diagnosis of gestational diabetes mellitus: a Jammu cohort study. J Assoc Physicians India. 2013;61:558-9.

15. Badikillaya VU, Adusumalli P, Venkata RG, et al. Effectiveness of Diabetes in Pregnancy Study Group India (DIPSI) diagnostic criterion in detecting gestational diabetes mellitus—a pilot study in a rural population. Indian J Basic Appl Med Res. 2013;2(6):614-8.
16. Mohan V, Mahalakshmi MM, Bhavadharini B, et al. Comparison of screening for gestational diabetes mellitus by oral glucose tolerance tests done in the non-fasting (random) and fasting states. Acta Diabetol. 2014;51:1007-13.
17. WHO. Definition, diagnosis and classification of diabetes mellitus and its complications: report of a WHO consultation. Part 1, Diagnosis and classification of diabetes mellitus. Geneva: World Health Organization; 1999. p. 59.
18. World Health Organization. Diagnostic criteria and classification of hyperglycaemia first detected in pregnancy. Geneva: World Health Organization; 2013. pp. 1-63.

CHAPTER 7

Exploring Causes of Stillbirth in Diabetic Pregnancies

Kanwal Gujral, Sakshi Nayar

INTRODUCTION

Global prevalence of pregestational diabetes and gestational diabetes has increased in both high-income and low-income group countries.[1,2] Seshiah et al., have reported an overall gestational diabetes mellitus (GDM) burden in India at 13.9%, with higher prevalence in obese and urban women.[3]

Both pregestational (type I and II) and gestational diabetes contribute to perinatal mortality rate (PNMR) as indicated by the following data.

Type I diabetes—threefold to fivefold increase in stillbirths, 75% due to congenital malformations and preterm births.[4] Meta-analysis of 33 studies comparing outcomes in type I and type II diabetes has reported higher PNMR in type II as compared to type I diabetes [odds ratio (OR), 1.5; 95% confidence interval (CI), 1.15–1.98].[5] Cundy et al. in an observational study in Auckland have reported PNMR as:

- Type I diabetes mellitus (type I DM)—12.5/1,000 live borns
- Type II diabetes mellitus (type II DM)—46.1/1,000 live borns
- GDM—8.9/1,000 live borns.

Overall there was sevenfold increase in late fetal deaths, 2.5-fold increase in intermediate fetal and late neonatal deaths. Many GDM were diagnosed as type II diabetes later.[6]

Study from England, Wales, and Northern Ireland has reported PNMR at 31.8/1,000 live borns which is four times higher than general population.[7]

Exploring causes of stillbirth in diabetic pregnancies is a challenging task. About 50% of stillbirths are due to associated conditions such as superimposed preeclampsia, fetal growth restriction (FGR), congenital malformation, abruptio placenta, intrauterine infections, diabetic ketoacidosis, and birth asphyxia.

Superimposed preeclampsia or hypertension can cause impedance in uteroplacental circulation leading to FGR, chronic fetal hypoxia, and fetal death. Placental abruption because of sudden rise in blood pressure (BP) can be another additive factor. Diabetic women with vascular complications can manifest FGR as early as in second trimester.

Diabetic ketoacidosis complicates 0.5–3% of pregnancies and can cause sudden fetal death if not promptly corrected. Possible explanation is a sudden reduction in uteroplacental flow and fetal oxygenation. Maternal severe hypoglycemia though often blamed can very occasionally result in fetal death.

Congenital fetal malformations are twofold to sixfold higher in type I and type II diabetic mothers.[2,4,7] The associated anomalies are of central nervous system (anencephaly, meningomyelocele, and encephalocele), cardiovascular system (atrial septal defect, ventricular septal defect, transposition of great arteries, and hypoplastic left heart), skeletal system (caudal regression syndrome), renal (agenesis and polycystic kidneys), and gastrointestinal (anorectal and duodenal malformation). Pre- and periconceptional hemoglobin A1c (HbA1c) level correlates with fetal anomalies, incidence being same as nondiabetic pregnancies at HbA1c less than 7.5% and 22% at HbA1c of 10. With advances in ultrasound majority of anomalies can be detected at midtrimester scan and pregnancies terminated resulting in fewer antepartum deaths. However, malformations are important contributors to neonatal deaths.

It is important to remember that in about 50% of cases, no cause is found, the so-called "unexplained ones". However, a constant link between maternal hyperglycemia and stillbirths has been established.[8,9]

Why and how stillbirth occurs is discussed here.

MATERNAL HYPERGLYCEMIA AND STILLBIRTH

Maternal hyperglycemia results in fetal hyperglycemia, which stimulates fetal pancreatic β-cells leading to marked fetal hyperinsulinemia. This results in accelerated fetal growth, excess subcutaneous fat, and increased hepatic glycogen. The increased fetal metabolism leads to increased tissue oxygen consumption, hypoxia, and finally fetal death. An association of fetal hyperglycemia, hyperinsulinemia, and chronic hypoxemia has been proven in animal studies.[10] Villous edema seen in the placentae of diabetic pregnancies can also impair oxygen transport resulting in fetal hypoxemia.

FETAL ERYTHROPOIETIN AND STILLBIRTH

Hypoxia stimulates erythropoietin (EP) synthesis. Recently it has been reported that amniotic fluid (AF) EP level is elevated prior to fetal death.[11] The AF EP level correlates with fetal plasma EP level.[12,13] Higher maternal glycosylated HbA1c level is also associated with higher EP level in umbilical venous sample. Widans et al suggest that insulin alone can exert a direct effect on fetal oxygenation because AF insulin level correlate with fetal EP level irrespective of glycemic status.[14] Teramo et al. have reported mean EP level at 14.0 μ/mL in diabetic pregnancies as against 6.3 μ/mL in nondiabetic pregnancies. Also AF EP level independently correlated with low umbilical pH and partial pressure of oxygen (PO_2). This implies that high EP levels can identify fetuses at risk of death or severe morbidity.[15] Elevated fetal EP levels can lead to neonatal polycythemia, stroke, seizures, and sudden death.

FETAL CARDIAC DYSFUNCTION AND STILLBIRTH

A link between cardiac dysfunction and stillbirth in pregnancy complicated with diabetes has been suggested. Hyperglycemia, hyperinsulinemia, and increased fetal EP have a negative effect on fetal heart as depicted by ST changes on fetal electrocardiography (ECG) and abnormal fetal heart rate pattern in labor.[12,13,16]

B type natriuretic peptide (BNP/pro-BNP), which is a marker of cardiac stress, is increased in patients with cardiomyopathy, heart failure, severe fetal distress, children with congenital heart disease, and fetuses with septal hypertrophy.[17] A higher BNP level has been reported in fetal umbilical cord and neonatal plasma in diabetic pregnancies as compared to nondiabetic pregnancies.[18]

Troponin T level which indicates acute myocardial damage is also seen to be elevated in umbilical cord of newborn with septal hypertrophy.[19] Russel et al., in a study of 45 women with type I diabetes have reported both troponin and BNP to be higher in neonates with clinically diagnosed cardiomyopathy. Pro-BNP correlated with interventricular septum thickness.[20]

It has been observed that about 40% of diabetic infants have septal hypertrophy and cardiomyopathy.

OXIDATIVE STRESS AND STILLBIRTH

Oxidative stress either by increased generation of free radicals or by inadequate antioxidant defense can lead to abnormal cardiac remodeling, hypertrophic cardiomyopathy, and fetal death.[21] Sarikabadayi et al. in a prospective study of umbilical cord levels of TOS (total oxidant status), OSI (oxidative stress index), and TAC (total antioxidant capacity) have reported significantly higher levels of TOS and OSI in diabetic pregnancies whether on insulin or diet as compared to nondiabetic pregnancies ($p \leq 0.001$). TAC levels were similar in all three groups. Maternal HbA1c levels correlated with TOS and OSI.[22]

Topcuoglu et al. have reported increased levels of OSI and TOS in diabetic pregnancies despite compensatory increase in TAC. Both OSI and TOS correlated with thickening of interventricular septum, HbA1c, and hematological involvement in first 3 days of life.[23]

From the above data, it is clear that hyperglycemia is the real culprit in causing fetal mortality through a variety of pathways. The pathogenesis of stillbirth in diabetes is summarized in Flowchart 7.1.

Flowchart 7.1: Pathogenesis of stillbirth in diabetes.

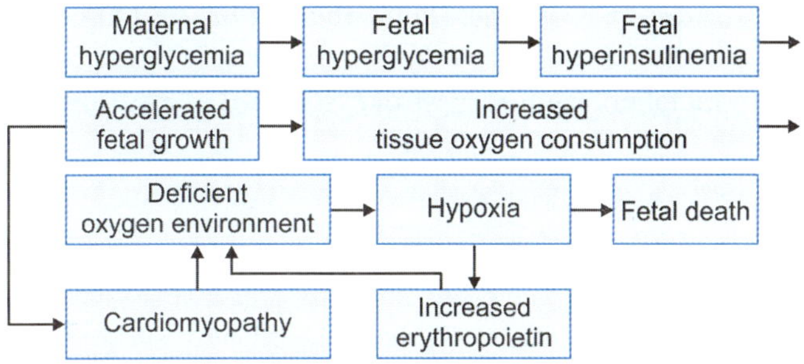

CONCLUSION

Some of the strategies to prevent stillbirth are involvement of a multi-disciplinary team consisting of an obstetrician, a physician/endocrinologist, neonatologist, dietician, and physical instructor for the management of a diabetic pregnancy. Preconceptional optimization of glycemic status, pre-conceptional folic acid supplementation, strict glycemic control through each trimester, regular fetal surveillance, and timely intervention are important measures which would optimize fetomaternal outcome.

KEY POINTS

- Both pregestational (type I and II) and gestational diabetes contribute to perinatal mortality rate (PNMR).
- About 50% of stillbirths are due to associated conditions such as superimposed preeclampsia, fetal growth restriction (FGR), congenital malformation, abruptio placenta, intrauterine infections, diabetic keto-acidosis, and birth asphyxia.
- Congenital fetal malformations are twofold to sixfold higher in type I and type II diabetic mothers.
- Diabetic ketoacidosis, hypoglycemia may cause a stillbirth but approximately 50% are unexplained.
- An association of maternal hyperglycemia with fetal hyperglycemia, hyperinsulinemia, chronic hypoxemia and finally death may be present.
- Chronic hypoxia state in the fetus of diabetic pregnancy increases fetal EP which has a negative effect on fetal heart. BNP is also high in diabetic pregnancies. These may cause cardiac dysfunction.
- Increased oxidative stress in diabetic pregnancy is associated with thickening of interventricular septum, HbA1c, and hematological involve ment which may be detrimental for the fetus.
- Preconceptional optimization of glycemic status, preconceptional folic acid supplementation, strict glycemic control through each trimester,

regular fetal surveillance, and timely intervention are important measures which would optimize fetomaternal outcome.

REFERENCES

1. Anna V, van der Ploeg HP, Cheung NW, et al. Sociodemographic correlates of the increasing trend in prevalence of gestational diabetes mellitus in a large population of women between 1995 and 2005. Diabetes Care. 2008;31:2288-93.
2. Bell R, Bailey K, Cresswell T, et al. Trends in prevalence and outcomes of pregnancy in women with pre-existing type I and type II diabetes. BJOG. 2008;115:445-52.
3. Seshiah V, Balaji V, Balaji MS, et al. Pregnancy and diabetes scenario around the world: India. Int J Gynaecol Obstet. 2009;104:S35-8.
4. Dudley DJ. Diabetic-associated stillbirth: incidence, pathophysiology and prevention. Obstet Gynecol Clin North Am. 2007;34:293-307.
5. Balsells M, Garcia-Patterson A, Gich I, et al. Maternal and fetal outcome in women with type 2 versus type 1 diabetes mellitus: a systemic review and meta-anlysis. J Clin Endocrinol Metab. 2009;94:4284-91.
6. Cundy T, Gamble G, Townend K, et al. Perinatal mortality in type 2 diabetes mellitus. Diabet Med. 2000;17:33-9.
7. Macintosh MCM, Flemming KM, Bailey JA, et al. Perinatal mortality and congenital anomalies in babies of women with type 1 and type 2 diabetes in England, Wales and Northern Ireland: population based study. BMJ. 2006;333:177-82.
8. Lauenborg J, Mathiesen E, Ovesen P, et al. Audit on stillbirths in women with pre-gestational type 1 diabetes. Diabetes Care. 2003;26:1385-9.
9. Hanson U, Persson B. Outcome of pregnancies complicated by type 1 insulin-dependent diabetes in Sweden: acute pregnancy complications, neonatal mortality and morbidity. Am J Perinatol. 1993;10:330-3.
10. Philips AF, Dublin JW, Matty PJ, et al. Arterial hypoxemia and hyperinsulinemia in the chronically hyperglycaemic fetal lamb. Pediatr Res. 1982;16:653-8.
11. Buescher U, Hertwig K, Wolf C, et al. Erythropoietin in amniotic fluid as a marker of chronic fetal hypoxia. Int J Gynaecol Obstet. 1998;60:257-63.
12. Salvesen DR, Brudenell JM, Snijders RJ, et al. Fetal plasma erythropoietin in pregnancies complicated by maternal diabetes mellitus. Am J Obstet Gynecol. 1993;168: 88-94.
13. Teramo KA, Widness JA, Clemons GK, et al. Amniotic fluid erythropoietin correlates with umbilical plasma erythropoietin in normal and abnormal pregnancy. Obstet Gynecol. 1987;69:710-6.
14. Widness JA, Teramo KA, Clemons GK, et al. Direct relationship of antepartum glucose control and fetal erythropoietin in human type 1 (insulin-dependent) diabetic pregnancy. Diabetologia. 1990;33:378-83.
15. Teramo K, Kari MA, Eronene M, et al. High amniotic fluid erythropoietin levels are associated with an increased frequency of fetal and neonatal morbidity in type 1 diabetic pregnancies. Diabetologia. 2004;47:1695-703.
16. Yli BM, Kallen K, Stray-Pedersen B, et al. Intrapartum fetal ECG and diabetes. J Matern Fetal Neonatal Med. 2008;21:231-8.
17. de Lemos JA, McGuire DK, Drazner MH. B-type natriuretic peptide in cardiovascular disease. Lancet. 2003;362:316-22.
18. Girsen A, Ala-Kopsala M, Makikallio K, et al. Increased fetal cardiac natriuretic peptide secretion in type-1 diabetic pregnancies. Acta Obstet Gynecol Scand. 2008; 87:307-12.

19. Fleming SM, O'Gorman T, O'Btyne L, et al. Cardiac troponin I and N-terminal pro-brain natriuretic peptide in umbilical artery blood in relation to fetal heart abnormalities during labor. Pediatr Cardiol. 2001;22:393-6.
20. Russell NE, Higgins MF, Amaruso M, et al. Troponin T and pro-B-type natriuretic peptide in fetuses of type 1 diabetic mothers. Diabetes Care. 2009;32:2050-5.
21. Lappas M, Hiden U, Desoye G, et al. The role of oxidative stress in the pathophysiology of gestational diabetes mellitus. Antioxid Redox Signal. 2011;15:3061-100.
22. Sarikabadayi YU, Aydemir O, Aydemir C, et al. Umbilical cord oxidative stress in infants of diabetic mothers and its relation to maternal hyperglycemia. J Pediatr Endocrinol Metab. 2011;24:671-4.
23. Topcuoglu S, Karatekin G, Yavuz T, et al. The relationship between the oxidative stress and the cardiac hypertrophy in infants of diabetic mothers. Diabtes Res Clin Pract. 2015;109:104-9.

CHAPTER 8

Glycemic Goals and Monitoring Methods in Gestational Diabetes

Anupam Prakash

INTRODUCTION

Studies across the world have stressed upon the need to keep plasma sugar levels under control, more so during pregnancy. In fact, gestational diabetes mellitus is considered to be one of the conditions which require a "tight" glycemic control. By tight glycemic control is meant, a sufficient enough glycemic control so as to be able to prevent microvascular complications and simultaneously not cause hypoglycemia.[1] This needs to be individualized for each person. However, several studies over the turn of the 21st century including the landmark Diabetes Control and Complications Trial (DCCT) and United Kingdom Prospective Diabetes Study (UKPDS) studies gave a numerical value to this "tight" glycemic control, equating it to a glycosylated hemoglobin (A1c) of less than 7.0%. A tight glycemic control is well-accepted to reduce the risk of microvascular complications of diabetes, and if initiated early, may also help reduce macrovascular complications, though the latter benefits may take much longer to be evident. Various conditions that require tight glycemic control included diabetic nephropathy, postrenal transplant patients, and gestational diabetes mellitus.

GLYCEMIC GOALS IN GESTATIONAL DIABETES MELLITUS

Hyperglycemia in gestational diabetes mellitus is detrimental to the fetus as well as the mother. Gestational diabetes mellitus is now an established risk factor for future development of diabetes in the mother. Besides, it can result in adverse perinatal outcomes including large for gestational age babies, macrosomia, birth defects, stillbirths, neonatal hypoglycemia, and increased requirement of induction of labor and need for caesarean section, among others. Therefore, there is a definite need for adequate control of blood sugar during pregnancy. The glycemic targets in gestational diabetes mellitus are based on recommendations from the Fifth International Workshop—Conference on Gestational Diabetes Mellitus, and the following targets are recommended to be achieved for maternal capillary glucose concentrations:[2,3]

- Preprandial plasma glucose: ≤95 mg/dL
- 1-hour postprandial glucose: ≤140 mg/dL
- 2-hour postprandial glucose: ≤120 mg/dL.

In patients of pregestational diabetes mellitus preexisting type 1 or type 2 diabetes, who become pregnant, the optimal glycemic targets are:

- Premeal, bedtime, and overnight glucose between 60 mg/dL and 99 mg/dL
- Peak postprandial glucose between 110 mg/dL and 129 mg/dL, and
- A1c of <6.0%.

The physiologic alterations in pregnancy normally cause fasting hypoglycemia as a result of the insulin-independent glucose uptake by the placenta, but postprandial hyperglycemia results as a consequence of diabetogenic placental hormones. The "insulin resistance" worsens as pregnancy progresses to the second and the third trimester.

The American College of Obstetricians and Gynecologists (ACOG) recommends the following targets:

- Fasting plasma glucose: <90 mg/dL
- 1-hour postprandial glucose: <1–140 mg/dL
- 2-hour postprandial glucose: <120 mg/dL.

If the ACOG goals are not achieved without significant hypoglycemia, slightly relaxed goals are suggested by the American Diabetes Association (ADA):

- Fasting plasma glucose: <105 mg/dL
- 1-hour postprandial glucose: <155 mg/dL
- 2-hour postprandial glucose: <130 mg/dL.

The ADA further recommends the need to set targets according to clinical experience and need for individualization of the treatment.

It is pertinent to mention at this point of time that the words blood sugar and plasma sugar may have been used in this write-up interchangeably, but in essence, these refer to plasma sugar only. Most of the present day glucometers measure whole blood glucose, but are so calibrated to show equivalent values in plasma glucose. The advantages of blood sugar testing by glucometer are enlisted in Box 8.1.

Box 8.1: Advantages of glucometer testing.

- Practical
- Easy to perform
- Bedside/at doorstep
- Standardized
- Reliable
- Actionable
- Emergency/routine
- Painful, but less than venepuncture, especially when repetitive measurements done.

MONITORING METHODS

Several monitoring methods can be employed to check for plasma sugar values, in order to take appropriate measures to effectively control glycemia. These include testing for blood glucose (venous blood samples in laboratory, or bedside glucometer-based testing), urine sugar testing, A1c testing, and some novel minimally invasive or noninvasive methods.

Urine Glucose (Sugar) Testing

Urine sugar testing was used earlier, but is not accurate and relies upon the appearance of blood sugar in urine when the blood sugar threshold of 180 mg/dL is exceeded. In pregnancy, the renal threshold is lowered, and hence, urine sugar will be positive at a lower blood sugar level. There are logistic issues in collection of urine sample and moreover, with collection of a double-voided urine sample each time. With the easy availability of glucometers and increasing awareness, urine sugar monitoring has virtually become an obsolete method in present day practice. Urine ketone testing still retains a place since blood ketone levels are not routinely easily available, though again it requires intelligent interpretation by the treating doctor. However, gestational diabetes patients have very less propensity to develop ketosis.

Blood Glucose Measurements—Venous Blood and Self-monitoring of Blood Glucose or Self-monitoring of Plasma Glucose

Self-monitoring of plasma glucose (SMPG) is the commonly used and recommended monitoring tool, which can be performed using a hand-held glucometer device, since it is easy to perform, requires less expertise, can be done by the patient and her relative at home itself, is less painful, and less expensive than repeated venepunctures. Besides, the results of glucometers are quite accurate (though less valid than venepuncture blood reports). However, a word of caution needs to be mentioned here, that the venepuncture reports of plasma glucose would differ from the glucometer reports, though the latter measures capillary whole blood glucose, but shows the equivalent capillary plasma glucose values. This difference is because the venous plasma glucose values are lower than capillary plasma venous glucose values by about 8–12% in the fasting state, and may be a little more in the postprandial state. Undoubtedly, SMPG is less painful than repeated venepunctures performed for venous blood sampling assessment, and does not carry the risk of thrombophlebitis.

The exact cost-effectiveness of SMPG in aiding better glycemic control in gestational diabetes has not yet been evaluated. However, the general observations in type 2 diabetes individuals[4] indicates that SMPG promotes

Box 8.2: Guide to using SMPG (adapted from IDF publication).

1. Patients and/or their caregivers should have the knowledge, skills, and willingness to incorporate SMPG monitoring and therapy adjustment, in order to achieve treatment goals.
2. SMPG should be considered at the time of diagnosis to enhance the understanding of the disease (gestational diabetes) as part of individual's education and increasing the awareness levels, facilitating timely treatment initiation, and titration optimization.
3. SMPG can be used as part of ongoing self-management education to assist patients to better understand their disease and provide means to actively and effectively participate in its control and treatment; by modifying behavioral and pharmacological interventions in consultation with their health care provider.
4. SMPG can help monitor impact of therapeutic decision-making.
5. Purpose of SMPG use should be clear to the patient and the health care provider, and mutually-agreed. The goals of SMPG and actual review should be documented.

(SMPG: Self-monitoring of plasma glucose; IDF: International Diabetes Federation)

better glycemia only if implemented together with training that includes learning how to adjust diet and lifestyle based on SMPG results. Also, in periods of rapid intensification, SMPG may have only limited impact. Thirdly, in patients with near-target metabolic control, SMPG had little effect. A guide to using SMPG has been reported by the International Diabetes Federation (IDF) for type 2 diabetes patients,[4] and is presented in Box 8.2 the same guide adapted and as applicable to gestational diabetes patients (Box 8.2). This may serve as the basis of how SMPG can be adopted in gestational diabetes mellitus individualizing the monitoring in these patients (determining the intensity and frequency).

The aim is to have plasma glucose levels within the target range throughout the 24-hour period. The nearest approximation can be from an 8-point or 9-point profile on SMPG which is performed before and 1-hour or 2-hour after the three major meals (breakfast, lunch, and dinner), at bedtime and at 3 am, and occasionally fasting blood sugar the next day morning. 1-hour postmeal blood glucose is preferred to 2-hour postmeal blood glucose, since controlling the former correlates with fewer chances of macrosomia, and better obstetric outcomes. Besides, women are reportedly more comfortable performing 1-hour postmeal blood glucose measurements.[3] SMPG should be performed on 3 days in a week, and the average prebreakfast values or average postprandial values can help in guiding behavioral changes, lifestyle/activity modifications and pharmacotherapeutic titrations. However, an 8-point profile on 3 days a week is a costly and painful exercise, requiring great motivation on the part of the patient, and willingness on the part of the treating doctor to be interpreting the results. Moreover, there should definitely exist a justified need for an intensive SMPG (Table 8.1), like if there is a requirement for intensification of treatment. A 7-point profile

Table 8.1: Focused/intensive self-monitoring of plasma glucose (SMPG) regimens.

7-point SMPG profile

	Prebreakfast	Postbreakfast	Prelunch	Postlunch	Predinner	Postdinner	Bedtime
Saturday	X	X	X	X	X	X	X
Sunday	X	X	X	X	X	X	X
Monday	X	X	X	X	X	X	X
Tuesday							
Wednesday							
Thursday							
Friday							

5-point SMPG profile

	Prebreakfast	Postbreakfast	Prelunch	Postlunch	Predinner	Postdinner	Bedtime
Saturday							
Sunday							
Monday	X	X		X	X	X	
Tuesday	X	X		X	X	X	
Wednesday	X	X		X	X	X	
Thursday							
Friday							

Staggered SMBG regimen

	Prebreakfast	Postbreakfast	Prelunch	Postlunch	Predinner	Postdinner	Bedtime
Saturday	X	X					
Sunday			X	X			
Monday					X	X	
Tuesday	X	X					
Wednesday			X	X			
Thursday					X	X	
Friday	X	X					

(excluding the 3.00 am or 4.00 am assessment), once a week or once a fortnight may be sufficient in most cases. Such a 7-point profile (Table 8.1) can be obtained as a staggered profile over a week as well. Alternatively, a 5-point SMPG profile (prebreakfast, postbreakfast, postlunch, predinner, and postdinner) may also be more focused in some cases, since postbreakfast and prelunch timings may not be much separated in time for some patients. A less intensive SMPG profiling (Table 8.2) may include premeal and postmeal testing in relation to only one meal in a day, covering different meals through the course of the week.

The time points when to perform SMPG and the intensity of SMPG monitoring depend upon various factors and need to be individualized for each patient of gestational diabetes. SMPG does make the patient more aware, and also acts as positive reinforcement for the patient. SMPG is considered to be an important self-management tool, only when the results are reviewed and acted upon by health care providers and/or people with diabetes, to actively modify behavior and/or adjust treatment.

Glycosylated Hemoglobin (A1c)

A1c may not be very useful during pregnancy, and is not preferred as a monitoring tool for gestational diabetes.[5] There is an increased red blood cell (RBC) turnover in pregnancy, which is responsible for a lower A1c during pregnancy.

As is a well-known fact, A1c represents the average glycemia over the preceding 3 months, and therefore, is not the primary glycemic target used to monitor glycemic control in gestational diabetes. A1c can however, be used as a secondary target [after self-monitoring of blood glucose (SMBG)], and needs to be performed monthly. A1c alone has a minimal role in management of gestational diabetes. The recommended target for A1c in gestational diabetes mellitus is 6.0–6.5%, less than 6.0% is optimal, as pregnancy progresses, to be achieved without hypoglycemia.

Newer Options

International Diabetes Federation states that continuous glucose monitoring can add an extra dimension to glycemia monitoring, and helps in identifying periods of unexpected hypoglycemia and hyperglycemia. Presently, the continuous glucose monitoring (CGM) devices are not being used in gestational diabetes,[5] and the recent availability of ambulatory glucose profile (AGP) by the flash glucose monitoring system developed by Abbot® (Fig. 8.1) utilizes a sensor which is a coin-sized disk-shaped device placed on the subject, and a reader which reads the blood glucose values, which can subsequently be transmitted to the computer for detailed analysis. The AGP is presently not standardized during pregnancy, and can at best be considered

Table 8.2: Low intensity self-monitoring of plasma glucose (SMPG) regimen.

Meal-based testing							
	Prebreakfast	*Postbreakfast*	*Prelunch*	*Postlunch*	*Predinner*	*Postdinner*	*Bedtime*
Saturday	X	X					
Sunday							
Monday			X	X			
Tuesday							
Wednesday					X	X	
Thursday							
Friday							

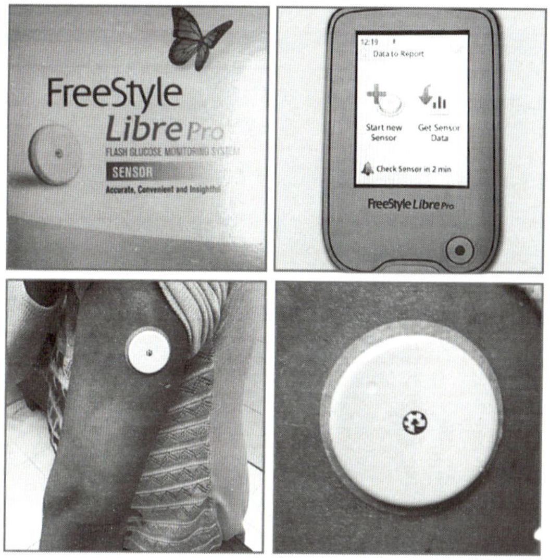

Fig. 8.1: Ambulatory glucose profile (AGP). Sensor device placed on a patient with a hand-held reader in the doctor's hand. *(for color version see Plate 1)*

to be a research instrument which can be utilized for monitoring glycemia in gestational diabetes and guiding patients' diet, lifestyle, and medication titration. The AGP records interstitial plasma glucose every 15 minutes for a period of 14 days, and can be a very helpful aid in detecting asymptomatic hypoglycemia and hyperglycemia events. Another important feature is that its application is virtually painless, and obviates need for repeated needle pricks for glycemic monitoring up to the time it is applied (14 days) on the patient. One sensor which records for a maximum period of 14 days in single application costs Rs. 1600-1900/-. The report format is displayed in Figure 8.2. Unlike the CGM devices which show a trend, the value can be read by the patient herself, and also show up an alarm if hypoglycemia occurs, the AGP device has to be read on a handheld reader, which presently has to be done at the level of the doctor. CGM devices are not commonly used with Gestational diabetes, and even with type 2 diabetes, since most of the patients would not be on insulin at such a young age. However, some type 1 diabetes patients specially the brittle diabetes patients, may be using insulin pumps, wherein the CGM devices would be in place, and so the reader needs to be aware of these.

Noninvasive and painless monitoring devices are being developed which can be used for glycemic monitoring. The GlucoWatch biographer is worn like a wristwatch, and measures glucose every 10 minutes through the skin. It is the first noninvasive glucose monitor, and uses an autosensor, a replaceable patch which sticks to the back of the watch, is adhesive to the skin and draws electric charge, which brings glucose to the skin and an enzyme

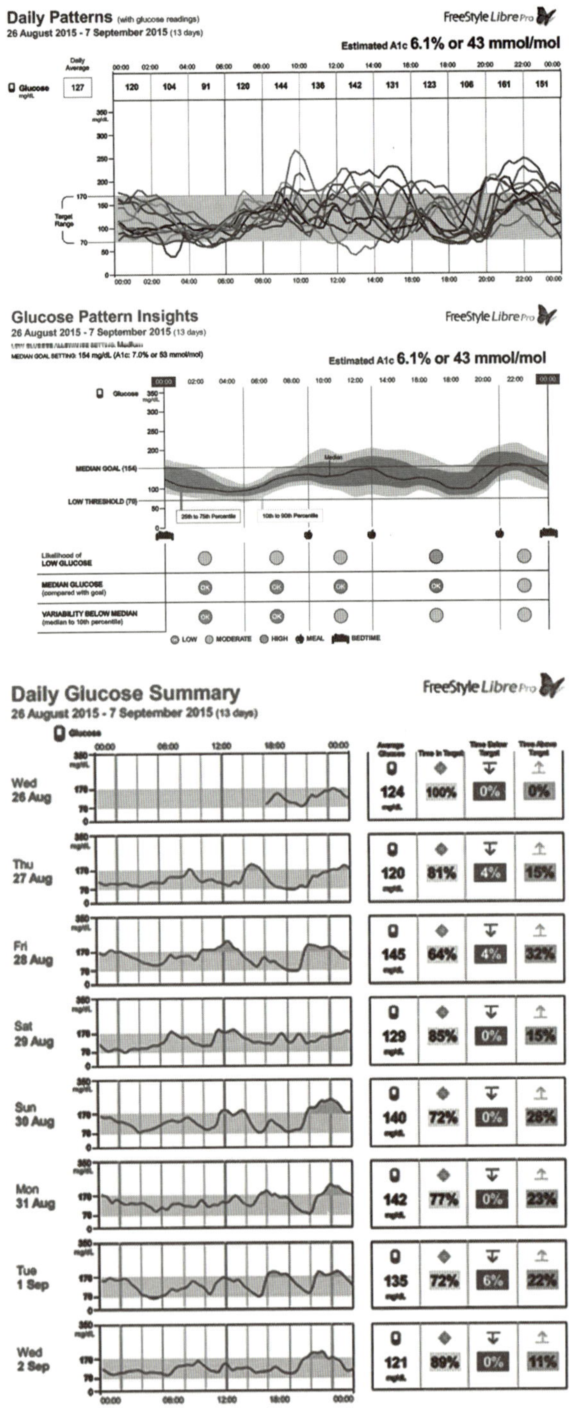

Fig. 8.2: Patterns obtained on 14 day Ambulatory Glucose Profile in addition to absolute values. *(for color version see Plate 2)*

reaction then estimates glucose with accuracy. The Silicon Microneedle (uses silicon microneedles and draws one-hundredth of a blood drop) and the Cell Robotics Lasette (uses laser technique to draw miniscule blood amount) are also virtually painless techniques for glucose monitoring. However, these are yet not easily accessible to the patients and wait testing in various clinical settings.

KEY POINTS

- Hyperglycemia in gestational diabetes can be detrimental to the fetus as well as the mother.
- The glycaemic targets (capillary glucose measurements) in pregnancy should be- fasting <90 mg/dL, 1 hour post-prandial glucose < 130–140 mg/dL and 2-hour post-prandial glucose <120 mg/dL.
- Glycemic control should be achieved without significant hypoglycemia. 1-hour post-prandial glucose levels are considered to be better than 2-hour post-prandial glucose levels, since are associated with less chances of macrosomia and better obstetric outcomes.
- Self-monitoring of plasma glucose with a glucometer is the most convenient and best suited technique for glycemic monitoring. Intensive regimens like the 7-point profile can be used to gauge adequate glycemic control.
- Urine sugar testing is not recommended.
- Glycosylated hemoglobin (A1c) has its own fallacies, needs to be performed monthly, and is ideally not recommended for glycemic monitoring. If at all A1c is used, SMBG still needs to be performed. Serum fructosamine is not recommended at present for glycemic monitoring.
- Newer continuous glucose monitoring (CGM) and ambulatory glucose profile (AGP) measurement techniques may help detect asymptomatic hypoglycemia and hyperglycemia episodes without the need for additional needle pricks, but these are not recommended as a routine for glycemic monitoring.

REFERENCES

1. Clement M, Bhattacharyya O, Conway JR. Is tight glycaemic control in type 2 diabetes really worthwhile? Yes. Can Fam Physician. 2009;55:580-82.
2. Management of Diabetes in Pregnancy. Diabetes Care. 2015:38(Suppl. 1):S77-9.
3. IDF Clinical Guidelines Task Force. Global Guideline on Pregnancy and Diabetes. Brussels: International Diabetes Federation, 2009, pp.1-32.
4. Self Monitoring of blood glucose in non-insulin treated Type 2 diabetes. Brussels: International Diabetes Federation, 2009, pp.1-39.
5. National Institute for Health and Care Excellence (NICE) Guideline. Diabetes in pregnancy: management from preconception to the postnatal period. www,nice.org.uk/guidance/ng3 Published: 25 February 2015. Accessed on 19th December, 2017.

CHAPTER 9

Medical Nutrition Therapy: Sheet Anchor in the Management of Gestational Diabetes Mellitus

Manju Puri, Vandana Mohan

INTRODUCTION

Gestational diabetes mellitus (GDM) is a common metabolic disorder among pregnant women. There has been a rapid rise in the prevalence of GDM and the newer diagnostic criteria has added to the burden.[1] Proper nutrition is of paramount importance for fetomaternal well-being during pregnancy, but the significance increases further in pregnant woman with GDM. GDM can be well-managed by a healthy balanced diet, physical activity, and appropriate pregnancy weight gain. Medical nutrition therapy (MNT) is the cornerstone of treatment for GDM.[2] With appropriate lifestyle modification, 70–85% of women with GDM can achieve adequate control of blood glucose without drug therapy.[3]

Pregnancy is a diabetogenic state consequent to insulin resistance due to hormones like human placental lactogen, progesterone, cortisol, and growth hormone. GDM develops when pancreas is not able to meet the increased demand of insulin during pregnancy leading to maternal hyperglycemia. GDM is associated with maternal and fetal complications. To maintain normoglycemia, lifestyle modification and pharmacological interventions are initiated in women with GDM. In majority of cases, lifestyle modifications alone in the form of MNT and exercise are sufficient to maintain normal blood glucose levels. This chapter will focus on the daily caloric requirement, caloric distribution across various meals, the glycemic status of various food, and monitoring women with GDM on MNT.

All women with GDM should be offered a proper dietary counseling at the time of diagnosis under a nutritional expert. The goals of dietary modifications in women with GDM as outlined by the American Congress of Obstetricians and Gynecologists (ACOG) in 2013 are to attain the desired level of glycemic control, provide adequate weight gain contributing to maternal and fetal well-being, and prevent the development of ketosis.[4]

DESIRED MATERNAL WEIGHT GAIN AND DAILY CALORIC REQUIREMENT

Maternal weight gain is a good indicator of nutritional status of mother and directly influences the birth weight of infant. Optimum weight gain during pregnancy is dependent on the maternal height and prepregnancy weight. The recommendations for optimum weight gain and caloric requirement based on the prepregnancy body mass index (BMI) of the pregnant woman according to latest American Diabetes Association (ADA) guidelines are as given in Table 9.1.[3]

The Western Pacific Regional Office (WPRO) of World Health Organization (WHO) proposed a specific classification in 2004 for obesity in Asian populations.[5] The definitions of normal, overweight, and obesity were defined as BMI in 18.5–22.9, 23–24.9, and more than and equal to 25 kg/m^2, respectively. The 2009 Institute of Medicine (IOM) guidelines for weight gain in twin pregnancy recommend BMI-specific weight gains for normal weight women of 17–25 kg (37–54 lb), overweight women of 14–23 kg (31–50 lb), and obese women of 11–19 kg (25–42 lb).[6] Monitoring the weight gain is important because excessive gain can cause fetal macrosomia, large for gestational age (LGA) babies, preterm delivery, and cesarean section.[7] In contrast, women who gain less weight have increased chances of small for gestational age (SGA) babies. Women with obesity should reduce their prepregnancy daily caloric consumption by about 30% while maintaining a minimum caloric intake of 1,600–1,800 kcal/kg/day.[8,9] Moreover, severe restriction of calories may lead to ketosis and therefore, weight loss is not recommended during pregnancy. Weekly weight checks are useful to monitor the weight gain.

Table 9.1: Recommendations for weight gain and calorie requirement in pregnancy.[3]

Prepregnancy BMI (kg/m^2)	*Total weight gain in kg (lb)*	*Rates of weight gain in second and third trimesters in lb/week (range)*	*Caloric requirements in kcal/kg/day*
Underweight (<18.5)	12.7–18.1 (28–40)	1 (1–1.3)	Up to 40
Normal weight (18.5–24.9)	11.3–15.9 (25–35)	1 (0.8–1)	30
Overweight (25.0–29.9)	6.8–11.3 (15–25)	0.6 (0.5–0.7)	22–25
Obese (≥30.0)	4.5–9.1 (10–20)	0.5 (0.4–0.6)	12–14

(BMI: Body mass index)

CALORIC DISTRIBUTION

The mainstay of MNT for women with GDM is proper distribution of calories with restriction of carbohydrates. According to ACOG 2013 guidelines, the recommended calorie distribution is: carbohydrate 33–40%, protein 20%, and fat 40%.[4] However, there is no robust evidence defining adequate proportion of carbohydrate in the diet of a GDM patient. The Endocrine Society suggests a lesser restrictive carbohydrate diet, comprising of 35–45% of total calories.[8] These recommendations are not rigid and the adjustment of carbohydrate consumption should be an ongoing process based on blood glucose levels, concentration of ketones, and weight gain of patient.[9]

The total calorie requirement should be distributed throughout the day, thus maintaining normal glucose levels. It is recommended that 10% of total calories are consumed at breakfast, 30% at lunch, 30% at dinner, and rest 30% divided at snacks. Carbohydrate should be evenly spread over each meal and snack. Proteins should be included with all meals to promote satiety. The dawn phenomenon is an unexplained rise in early morning blood sugar levels usually due to a previous night time rise of growth hormone which stimulates the liver to breakdown glycogen and release glucose into the bloodstream. As this phenomenon causes increase in early morning blood glucose levels, there is need to lower carbohydrate consumption at breakfast.

MEAL PLAN

The main idea of a meal plan is to maintain normal blood glucose levels throughout the day and avoid episodes of hyperglycemia and hypoglycemia. Frequent meals at an interval of two and half to three hours are advised. Ideally a daily meal plan for women with GDM should include three small to moderate sized meals along with two to four snacks. In order to prevent overnight ketosis, a small snack should be taken at bedtime.[9] Meal plans should take into consideration the cultural preferences, desired weight gain, and level of physical activity.[2]

GLYCEMIC STATUS OF FOOD ITEMS

It is not just the amount, the type of food is equally important. Complex carbohydrates are less likely to cause postprandial hyperglycemia and are therefore preferred over simple carbohydrates.[4] Foods with complex carbohydrates usually have a lower glycemic index (GI), and prevent sudden rise in postprandial blood glucose levels.

Glycemic index is a scientific ranking of how the foods we eat affect our blood glucose levels in postprandial period that is 2 or 3 hours after eating. Foods are measured against pure glucose, which has a value of 100 on the GI. The index ranges from 0 to 100. Accordingly, the foods are classified

Table 9.2: Classification of food items according to the glycemic index (GI).

	Low GI (0–55)	*Moderate GI (56–69)*	*High GI (70–100)*
Cereals and breads	Whole wheat bread/ roti, multigrain bread/roti, porridge, oat bran, spaghetti, rice noodles, macaroni, dalia, barley	Basmati rice, brown rice, pita bread, corn meal, whole white bread	White bread, tapioca, short grain white rice, sticky rice, corn flakes, bagel
Legumes and vegetables	All legumes/ lentils, cauliflower, cabbage, spinach, lettuce, broccoli, mushroom, onion, capsicum, brinjal, tomato, carrot, sweet potato, sweet corn	Canned potato, beetroot	Pumpkin, potato
Dairy	Milk, yoghurt, soya milk, custard	Full fat ice cream	
Fruits	Apple, pear, kiwi, oranges, grapes, peach, berries, coconut, nuts, raisins	Mango, banana, papaya	Watermelon, dates, lychees, pineapple

as high, medium, or low glycemic foods. The foods with high GI (70–100) breakdown quickly, release sugars rapidly into bloodstream, and cause rapid fluctuations in blood glucose levels. The foods with medium GI (56–69) breakdown moderately and release sugar moderately into bloodstream, whereas those with low GI (0–55) breakdown slowly, release sugars gradually into blood stream, and keep the blood glucose levels steady. Table 9.2 lists the commonly used food items according to the GI. Low GI foods are the best choice and should be ideally included in all meals.

Carbohydrates can be measured in terms of exchanges or portions that can be mixed and matched over meals (Box 9.1). The main meals should include 3–4 carbohydrate exchanges and 1–2 at snacks. (1 portion/exchange = 15 g of carbohydrate).

There are certain foods that contain very little carbohydrates and hence do not raise blood glucose levels. These are listed as below:

- *Fruits:* Lemon, lime, berries, and passion fruit. All other fruit contains carbohydrates.
- *Vegetables:* All salad and nonstarchy vegetables.

Box 9.1: Portion equivalent of various food items.

Cereals and grains
1 portion = 1 regular thin slice of bread, 2/3 cup cereal flakes, ¼ cup raw oats or muesli, ½ cup cooked pasta or noodles, 1/3 cup cooked rice, 2–3 plain biscuits or crackers, half roti.
Legumes and vegetables
1 portion = 1 medium potato, ½ cup mashed sweet potato or potato, ½ cup of corn, ½ cup legumes.
Fruits
1 portion = medium apple or orange or pear, ½ large banana, 2–3 plums or apricots or kiwi, ¾ cup diced or tinned fruit, 15–20 grapes or cherries, 1 tablespoon dried fruits, 125 mL juice.
Dairy products
1 portion = 1 cup milk, ½ tub fruit yoghurt (100 g), 1 tub natural or diet yoghurt (200g), ½ cup custard.

- *Protein foods:* Meat, chicken, fish, eggs, nuts, and cheese.
- *Fat-based foods:* Oils, margarine, peanut butter, avocado, mayonnaise, and salad dressings.

However, if eaten in large amounts, fat- or protein-based foods contribute to excess weight gain in pregnancy.

A diet with adequate dietary fiber, mainly cereals and fruits reduce the risk of developing GDM. Each 10 g/day increment in total fiber intake is associated with a 26% reduction in risk; each 5 g/day increment in cereal fiber and fruit fiber is associated with 23% and 26% reduction in GDM risk, respectively.[10] Increased dietary fiber intake reduces appetite and hence lower the total energy consumption. It also delays gastric emptying and slows glucose absorption leading to glucose homeostasis.[11] Some studies have shown a possible reduced incidence of GDM with the use of probiotics, most common being *Lactobacillus rhamnosus* and *Bifidobacterium lactis.*[10,12] Deficiency of vitamin D has also been implicated in the development of GDM. Vitamin D at normal levels (>30 ng/mL) is associated with a lower insulin resistance.[10] Myoinositol supplementation has been studied both as a potential treatment and prevention for GDM with insufficient evidence.[13,14] Carbohydrate foods that contain little nutritional value include soft drinks, fruit juice, lollies or sweets, chocolates, cakes, and biscuits and should be avoided.

Together with medical nutrition therapy, physical activity is a key component in the initial management of GDM. Physical activity improves insulin sensitivity and reduces both fasting and post prandial blood glucose concentrations in patients with diabetes. It also reduces or delays the need for insulin. There is no recommendation on any specific kind of exercise. The ADA, ACOG, and Endocrine Society guidelines recommend moderate exercise for 30 minutes most days of the week for women with GDM with no contraindication to physical activity.[4,8] The frequency to carry out exercises should be increased gradually to 45 min/day, five times a week.[15] Moderate exercises include brisk walking, recumbent bicycling, or 10 minutes of seated arm exercises after each meal. Even low-intensity exercise has shown benefits in mood, balance, back pain, and urinary incontinence.[16]

MONITORING AND FOLLOW-UP

Women with GDM should be advised to keep a record of all food and beverages consumed. This simple process helps in regulating caloric intake and rate of weight gain. It is a well-known behavioral tool that makes eating a more conscious behavior. The woman is asked to maintain food record for 3 days before seeking a diet plan from the dietician. It will help the dietician understand the food habits and plan a diet accordingly. Food records after education on the meal plan help practitioners assess patients' ability to follow the plan, acceptance of calorie level, and understanding of concept of MNT.

Once diagnosed with GDM, woman should start routine glucose monitoring. There is insufficient evidence regarding optimal frequency of testing. ACOG 2013 recommends glucose monitoring four times a day, fasting glucose and 1 or 2 hours after each meal.[4] There is no consensus on whether a 1-hour or a 2-hour postprandial reading is best. Self-monitoring of blood glucose (SMBG) allows women to become active participants in achieving euglycemia. Monitoring gives women immediate feedback about portion size, particular foods that cause hyperglycemia, stable temporal patterns of elevated blood glucose levels, and when in the day exercise is most likely to help keep blood glucose in the target range. SMBG helps the woman to tailor her meal and exercise plans to normalize blood glucose levels, and allows earlier introduction of insulin when necessary.

Regular testing for ketone in the urine is an inexpensive tool that gives objective information on actual caloric and carbohydrate intake. Measurement of prebreakfast urine ketone is recommended for patients on hypocaloric or carbohydrate- restricted diets. The persistence of small to moderate ketones indicate inadequate caloric intake, misunderstanding of the meal plan, or a woman secretly restricting food to avoid the addition of insulin.

It is estimated that 70–85% of cases of GDM can be controlled with lifestyle changes.[1,3] If the desired blood glucose levels are not achieved within 2 weeks, pharmacotherapy should be started.

ADA and ACOG target blood glucose levels are:

- Fasting blood glucose concentration ≤95 mg/dL (5.3 mmol/L)
- 1-hour postprandial blood glucose concentration ≤140 mg/dL (7.8 mmol/L)
- 2-hour postprandial glucose concentration ≤ 120 mg/dL (6.7 mmol/L).

Little guidance is available as to what proportion of measurements exceeding these thresholds should trigger intervention. Some suggest insulin for two or more elevated values in a 2-week interval, some initiate insulin when one-third of values exceed the target in a given week, while rest await more consistent elevations, especially if it is anticipated that further nutritional counseling may be effective.[17]

POSTPARTUM COUNSELING

After delivery, blood glucose levels usually return to normal. All women with GDM should have a glucose assessment to exclude ongoing hyperglycemia within 24–72 hours of delivery and before being discharged from hospital.[8,18] As GDM increases the chances of developing prediabetes or type 2 diabetes, a screening at 6–12 weeks postpartum using one-step approach (2-hour 75 g OGTT) is advised.[3,4] Women should be encouraged to achieve and maintain a healthy weight by lifestyle modifications and breast feeding that support weight loss after delivery with reduction in the risk of progression to type 2 diabetes later in life.[8,19] They are encouraged to follow a healthy well-balanced diet with plenty of fruits, vegetables, and whole grain cereals. Physical activity should be recommended.

Gestational diabetes mellitus is a disease with serious short-term and long-term consequences to the mother and the fetus. The incidence is on the rise due to high prevalence of overweight and obesity, coupled with sedentary lifestyle. It is recommended that all pregnant women are screened for GDM for an early detection and timely initiation of MNT to optimize perinatal outcome.

KEY POINTS

- Pregnancy is a diabetogenic state consequent to insulin resistance due to hormones.
- GDM can be well managed by a healthy balanced diet, physical activity, and appropriate pregnancy weight gain.
- MNT is the cornerstone of treatment for GDM.
- The goals of dietary modifications in women with GDM; to attain the desired level of glycemic control, provide adequate weight gain contributing to maternal and fetal well-being, and prevent the development of ketosis.
- Optimum weight gain during pregnancy is dependent on the maternal height and prepregnancy weight.
- The mainstay of MNT for women with GDM is proper distribution of calories with restriction of carbohydrates.
- The main idea of a meal plan is to maintain normal blood glucose levels throughout the day by 2–3 main meals and 2–4 small snacks.
- It is not just the amount, the type of food is equally important and carbohydrates with low GI are preferred.

- If the desired blood glucose levels; F > 95 mg/dL and 2-hour postprandial >120 mg/dL, are not achieved within 2 weeks, pharmacotherapy should be started.

REFERENCES

1. Bortolon LNM, Triz Lde PL, Faustino B de S, et al. Gestational Diabetes Mellitus: New Diagnostic criteria. Open J Endocr Metab Dis. 2016;6:13-9.
2. Metzger BE, Buchanan TA, Coustan DR. Summary and recommendations of the Fifth International Workshop—Conference on Gestational Diabetes Mellitus. Diabetes Care. 2007;30(2):251-60.
3. American Diabetes Association. Management of diabetes in pregnancy. Diabetes Care. 2016;39(1):94-8.
4. Committee on Practice Bulletins-Obstetrics. Practice Bulletin No. 137: Gestational diabetes mellitus. Obstet Gynecol. 2013;122:406-16.
5. WHO Expert Consultation. Appropriate body-mass index for Asian populations and its implications for policy and intervention strategies. Lancet. 2004;363:157-63.
6. Rasmussen KM, Yaktine AL. Weight Gain during Pregnancy: Reexamining the Guidelines. Washington (DC): Institute of Medicine (US) and National Research Council (US) and Committee to Reexamine IOM Pregnancy Weight Guidelines; 2009.
7. Cheng YW, Chung JH, Kurbisch-Block I, et al. Gestational weight gain and gestational diabetes mellitus: perinatal outcomes. Obstet Gynecol. 2008;112:1015-22.
8. Blumer I, Hadar E, Hadden DR, et al. Diabetes and pregnancy: An Endocrine Society clinical practice guideline. J Clin Endocrinol Metab. 2013;98:4227-49.
9. American Diabetes Association. Nutrition recommendations and interventions for diabetes: a position statement of the American Diabetes Association. Diabetes Care. 2008;31(1):61-78.
10. Gunasekaran PK. Changing Trends in Management of Gestational Diabetes Mellitus. World J Diabetes. 2015;6:284-95.
11. Zhang C, Liu S, Solomon CG, et al. Dietary fiber intake, dietary glycemic load, and the risk for gestational diabetes mellitus. Diabetes Care. 2006;29:2223-30.
12. Luoto R, Laitinen K, Nermes M, et al. Impact of maternal probiotic-supplemented dietary counselling on pregnancy outcome and prenatal and postnatal growth: a double-blind, placebo controlled study. Br J Nutr. 2010;103(12):1792-9.
13. Corrado F, D'Anna R, Di VG, et al. The effect of myoinositol supplementation on insulin resistance in patients with gestational diabetes. Diabet Med. 2011;28(8):972-5.
14. D'Anna R, Di BV, Rizzo P, et al. Myo-inositol may prevent gestational diabetes in PCOS women. Gynecol Endocrinol. 2012;28(6):440-2.
15. Padatachee C, Coombes J. Exercise Guidelines for Gestational Diabetes Mellitus. World J Diabetes. 2015;6:1033-44.
16. Kampmann U, Madsen LR, Skajaa GO, et al. Gestational diabetes: A clinical update. World J Diabetes. 2015;6:1065-72.
17. Whalen KL, Taylor JR. Gestational Diabetes Mellitus. In: Murphy JE, Lee MW (Eds). Pharmacotherapy Self-Assessment Program. Lenexa, KS: American College of Clinical Pharmacy; 2017. pp. 7-26.
18. National Collaborating Centre for Women's and Children's Health (UK). Diabetes in Pregnancy: Management of diabetes and its complications from preconception to the postnatal period. London: RCOG Press; 2008.
19. Garrison A. Screening, diagnosis, and management of gestational diabetes mellitus. Am Fam Physician. 2015;91:460-7.

CHAPTER 10

Physical Activity for Patients with Diabetes in Pregnancy: Clinical Update

Pikee Saxena, Rajiv Gupta

INTRODUCTION

With the changing lifestyles and the increase in the sedentary way of life, maintenance of physical health and activity has become an emerging challenge. For maintaining glucose homeostasis and overall health in individuals with diabetes and pre-diabetes, it is important to adopt and maintain physical activity. Physical activity is defined as any bodily movement produced by the contraction of skeletal muscles while exercise is physical activity consisting of planned, structured, and repetitive bodily movements done to improve one or more components of physical fitness.[1]

Although there is a concern regarding exercise for pregnant women, it has been observed that physical activity during uncomplicated pregnancy has minimal risks and may prevent both gestational diabetes (GDM) and possibly development of Type 2 diabetes mellitus later in life. Engaging in regular physical activity before pregnancy frequently has been associated with a reduced risk of developing obesity, increased weight gain during pregnancy, GDM and preeclampsia.[2] Most exercise recommendations for diabetic pregnancy are same as for normal pregnancy.

RECOMMENDATIONS BY DIFFERENT AUTHORITIES ON EXERCISE DURING PREGNANCY

The American College of Obstetricians and Gynecologists:[3]

In the absence of either medical or obstetric complications, moderate exercise for ≥30 minutes a day on most, if not all, days of the week is recommended for pregnant women.

The Society of Obstetricians and Gynaecologists of Canada[4]

All women without contraindications should be encouraged to participate in aerobic and strength-conditioning exercises as part of a healthy lifestyle during pregnancy.

Royal College of Obstetricians and Gynaecologists (United Kingdom)[5]

A review of the evidence suggests that, in most cases, exercise is safe for both mother and fetus during pregnancy. Women should therefore be encouraged to initiate or continue exercise to derive the health benefits associated with such activities.

The Royal Australian and New Zealand College of Obstetricians and Gynaecologists[6]

Moderate-intensity aerobic exercise is safe in pregnancy; for trained athletes, it may be possible to exercise at a higher level than is currently recommended. Among the numerous benefits of remaining active during pregnancy are, improved weight control and maintenance of fitness, as well as possible benefits in terms of reduced risk of development of gestational diabetes mellitus and improved psychological functioning.

The U.S. Department of Health and Human Services[7]

For healthy pregnant and postpartum women, the guidelines recommend at least 150 minutes per week of moderate-intensity aerobic activity (i.e., equivalent to brisk walking). This activity should be spread throughout the week and adjusted as medically indicated. The guidelines advise that pregnant women who habitually engage in vigorous-intensity aerobic activity (i.e., the equivalent of running or jogging) or who are highly active can continue physical activity during pregnancy and the postpartum period, provided that they remain healthy and discuss with their health care provider how and when activity should be adjusted over time.

RESPONSE OF THE FETUS TO MATERNAL EXERCISE

A number of studies have evaluated the effect of maternal exercise on fetal heart rate changes and birth weight. Studies have demonstrated minimum-to-moderate increases in fetal heart rate by 10–30 beats per minute over the baseline during or after exercise.[8-11] Three meta-analyses concluded that the differences in birth weight were minimal to none in women who exercised during pregnancy compared with controls.[12-14] However, women who continued to exercise vigorously during the third trimester were more likely to deliver infants weighing 200–400 g less than comparable controls, although there was not an increased risk of fetal growth restriction.[12-14] A cohort study that assessed umbilical artery blood flow, fetal heart rates, and biophysical profiles before and after strenuous exercise in the second trimester demonstrated that 30 minutes of strenuous exercise was well tolerated by women and fetuses in active and inactive pregnant women.[11]

BENEFITS OF EXERCISE DURING PREGNANCY

Physical activity performed during pregnancy benefits a woman's overall health. Pregnant women undertaking moderate intensity physical activity can maintain or increase their cardio respiratory fitness.[2] A maternal exercise program during pregnancy does not increase the risk of low birth weight, preterm delivery or early pregnancy loss. On the other hand, regular exercise reduces the risk of pregnancy complications such as preeclampsia, edema, constipation, backache, weight gain, GDM and during labor shortens the duration of active labor and helps in pain relief. In the postpartum period, exercise facilitates weight loss and postpones or prevents development of type 2 diabetes mellitus.

Recreational physical activity improves general wellbeing, maternal mood and mental health. Exercise improves insulin sensitivity and glucose clearance by a variety of mechanisms. On a molecular level, exercise is associated with increased expression of insulin signaling proteins and enzymes which participate in skeletal muscle and fat uptake of glucose. Bung et al.[15] investigated the use of exercise in women with GDM. Seventeen of the twenty-one women in the exercise group, who were all previously insulin dependent were able to maintain normal glucose levels without using insulin. Maternal complications did not differ between the exercise and control group. They concluded that exercise was safe and advantageous during pregnancy and helped to control blood sugar levels. Studies have shown that an exercise program initiated after the diagnosis of GDM may reduce the requirement for Insulin therapy and improve glycemic control in late pregnancy. In a recent clinical trial a moderate physical activity program performed thrice in a week during pregnancy was found to improve levels of maternal glucose tolerance in healthy, pregnant women.[16]

PHYSIOLOGICAL CHANGES IN PREGNANCY AFFECTING EXERCISE

During pregnancy the ligaments and joints become lax due to hormonal changes. Therefore jerky, high motion impact movements should be avoided to prevent injury. As pregnancy advances the diaphragm is pushed upwards by the enlarging uterus which reduces the respiratory volumes. During exercise, blood and oxygen is diverted to the exercising muscles which may compromise the oxygen supply to the fetus and other organs of the body.

In pregnant women, BMR is higher and during exercise temperature may rise leading to hyperthermia and dehydration. Due to the enlarging uterus, there is progressive lordosis. This may disturb the balance of the body and the woman is more prone to fall.

EXERCISES TO BE AVOIDED DURING PREGNANCY[2]

Avoid activity lying flat on the back and any exercise that increases the risk of falling or abdominal trauma e.g. contact or collision sports, horseback riding, water skiing, soccer, outdoor cycling, basketball, racquet sports, scuba diving, hot yoga.

CONTRAINDICATIONS TO EXERCISE DURING PREGNANCY[2]

If a pregnant woman has medical complications or contraindications, such as serious heart or lung disease, severe anemia, premature labor, threatened abortion, persistent bleeding during 2nd or 3rd trimester, placenta previa, incompetent os, ruptured membranes, preeclampsia, growth restricted fetus, chronic placental abruption, multiple pregnancy at risk of preterm labor, exercise should be avoided.

PRECAUTIONS TO BE TAKEN DURING EXERCISE

A woman not used to exercise before pregnancy should begin exercising in a carefully structured program under supervision of the obstetrician/physician and a qualified physical trainer.

If a woman has been doing weight bearing exercises before pregnancy, transition may be done from weight-bearing to non-weight bearing exercises with advancing pregnancy (e.g., cycling and swimming in the second half of pregnancy).

Collision sports and deep-water diving should be avoided.

If the pregnant woman exhibits symptoms such as dizziness, dyspnea, amniotic fluid leaking, vaginal bleeding, headache, chest pain, calf pain or swelling, they should stop exercise immediately and seek medical advice.

Warm up should be done before and after exercise.

Pregnant women should wear loose fitting clothes and comfortable footwear.

They should keep themselves well-hydrated before, during and after exercise.

Exercise should be done in an environment with appropriate temperature and humidity. Overheating should be avoided as hyperthermia has been linked to neural tube defects during the first trimester.

Breasts should be well supported during exercise, sports bra may be used. Comfortable, flat, without heel footwear should be used. Women should avoid exercising lying flat on their backs to avoid supine hypotension syndrome.

TYPE OF EXERCISE

A variety of exercises ranging from low exerting exercise such as yoga, aerobic classes, brisk walking, swimming etc. are safe for the mother and fetus.

Aerobic exercises should be preferred over resistance strength training unless the woman has been doing resistance strength training before pregnancy.

Yoga is an ancient mind-body practice that originated in India and is becoming increasingly popular worldwide as a health practice for a variety of immunological, neuromuscular, psychological, and pain conditions. It has the potential to create balance along emotional, mental, physical, and spiritual dimensions Yoga is a comprehensive system that uses physical postures (asana), breathing exercises (pranayama), concentration and meditation (dharana and dhyana), and contemplative practice.

Swimming in moderate intensity is considered useful as it tones the muscles, improves fitness, relieves backache and reduces the chances of fall and injury.

Aerobic exercise-walk, stationary cycle, swim, aquatic activities, conditioning machines, prenatal exercise classes, prenatal yoga, seated exercise, possible jogging and running (if highly active before pregnancy).

Resistance exercise-Light or Moderate resistance exercise

INTENSITY OF EXERCISE

During pregnancy, gradually increasing physical activity energy expenditure reduces the risk of GDM. If the exercise is vigorous, less duration of exercise is required. As blunted and normal heart-rate responses to exercise have been reported in pregnant women, the use of ratings of perceived exertion may be a more effective means to monitor exercise intensity during pregnancy than heart-rate parameters.[17] Using the "talk test" is another simple and practical way to measure exertion. As long as a woman can carry on a conversation while exercising, she is likely not overexerting herself.[18]

Frequency: 3-7 days spread throughout the week

Duration: 30 minutes/session on most if not all days of the week At least 150 minutes of moderate intensity spread throughout the week.

Progression: The woman should gradually increase the exercise duration and intensity if she has just started. If she has been active, pregnant woman should maintain or lower intensity of exercise during pregnancy.

Safety of exercise during pregnancy is of vital importance—A pre and post warm up exercise is beneficial as it helps the body to adjust with the changing physiological and mechanical demands.

A recent meta-analysis reported that pregnant women with GDM who exercised on a cycle or arm ergometer or performed resistant training three times a week for 20-45 minutes experienced better glycemic control, lower fasting and postprandial glucose levels and improved cardio respiratory fitness.[2]

EXERCISE DURING THE POSTPARTUM PERIOD

The postpartum period is the best time for the obstetrician to initiate, recommend, and reinforce a healthy lifestyle. Gradually after delivery, exercise activities should be resumed or new exercise schedule should be initiated which should continue throughout life. Exercise in the postpartum period should be tailored depending on the mode of delivery-vaginal or cesarean and associated medical or surgical complications.

Deep breathing, simple leg movement exercise and pelvic floor exercises may be initiated soon after delivery. Women should take healthy nutritious diet and keep themselves well-hydrated during exercise in the postpartum period. Frequent breast feeding and breast support will prevent breast discomfort during this time.

Several reports indicate that women's level of participation in exercise programs diminishes after childbirth, frequently leading to overweight and obesity.[19,20] Regular aerobic exercise in lactating women has been shown to improve maternal cardiovascular fitness without affecting milk production, composition, or infant growth.

CONCLUSION

For the overall management of health and the glycemic control in pregnant women with diabetes, it is important to include physical activity and exercise in their daily schedule. Precautions should be taken in case the pregnant woman is suffering from medical or obstetrical health complications. Therefore, it is important that all the physical activities and exercise be tailored according to the specific needs and requirements. Behavioral changes and lifestyle modifications initiated during pregnancy should be continued after delivery to avoid or delay development of recurrent GDM, diabetes, obesity later in life.

KEY POINTS

- Women with uncomplicated pregnancy should participate in regular aerobic and strength conditioning exercise.
- Exercise during pregnancy does not cause any potential harm to the mother or fetus. It has several benefits like it reduces the risk of preeclampsia, edema, constipation, backache, weight gain, GDM. During labor it helps to shorten the duration of active labor.
- In the postpartum period, exercise facilitates weight loss and postpones or prevents development of type 2 diabetes mellitus.
- Assessment of medical and obstetric risks should be undertaken to identify potential contraindications to exercise for the pregnant woman prior to commencing an exercise program.
- Obstetrician and physical trainer should help to decide about the type of exercise, frequency, duration and intensity of exercise.

REFERENCES

1. American College of Sports Medicine. ACSM's guidelines for exercise testing and prescription. 9th ed. Philadelphia (PA): Wolters Kluwer/Lippincott Williams & Wilkins; 2014.
2. Ceysens G, Rouiller D, Boulvain M: Exercise for diabetic pregnant women. Cochrane Database Sys Rev. 2006;(3):CD0004225.
3. Physical activity and exercise during pregnancy and the postpartum period ACOG Committee Obstetric Practice: ACOG Committee opinion: Number 650, December 2015. Available at https://www.acog.org/Clinical-Guidance-and-Publications/Committee-Opinions/Committee-on-Obstetric-Practice/Physical-Activity-and-Exercise-During-Pregnancy-and-the-Postpartum-Period. Accessed on 4/1/18.
4. Davies GA1, Wolfe LA, Mottola MF, et al. Society of Obstetricians and gynecologists of Canada, SOGC Clinical Practice Obstetrics Committee. Joint SOGC/CSEP clinical practice guideline: exercise in pregnancy and the postpartum period. Can J Appl Physiol. 2003;28(3):330-41.
5. Royal College of Obstetricians and Gynaecologists: RCOG Statement No. 4: Exercise in pregnancy. Royal College of Obstetricians and Gynaecologists, January 1, 2006. Available at: http:// www.rcog.org.uk/womens health/ clinical-guidance/exercise-pregnancy. Accessed on 4.1.18
6. Exercise during pregnancy. Available at https://www.ranzcog.edu.au/RANZCOG_SITE/media/RANZCOG-MEDIA/Women's%20Health/Statement%20and%20guidelines/Clinical-Obstetrics/Exercise-during-pregnancy-(C-Obs-62)-New-July-2016.pdf?ext=.pdf .Accessed on 4.1.18.
7. Department of Health and Human Services. 2008 physical activity guidelines for Americans. Washington, DC: DHHS; 2008. Available at: http://health.gov/paguidelines. Accessed on 4.1.18.
8. Carpenter MW, Sady SP, Hoegsberg B, et al. Fetal heart rate response to maternal exertion. JAMA 1988;259:3006-9.
9. Wolfe LA, Lowe-Wyldem SJ, Tanmer JE, McGrath MJ. Fetal heart rate during maternal static exercise. Can J Sport Sci 1988;13:95-6.
10. Artal R, Rutherford S, Romem Y, et al. Fetal heart rate responses to maternal exercise. Am J Obstet Gynecol. 1986;155:729-33.
11. Szymanski LM, Satin AJ. Exercise during pregnancy: fetal responses to current public health guidelines. Obstet Gynecol. 2012;119:603-10.
12. Kramer MS, McDonald SW. Aerobic exercise for women during pregnancy. Cochrane Database of Systematic Reviews 2006, Issue 3. Art. No.: CD000180. DOI: 10.1002/14651858.CD000180.
13. Lokey EA, Tran ZV, Wells CL, et al. Effects of physical exercise on pregnancy outcomes: a meta-analytic review. Med Sci Sports Exerc. 1991;23:1234-9.
14. Leet T, Flick L. Effect of exercise on birthweight. Clin Obstet Gynecol. 2003;46:423-31.
15. Bung P, Artal R, Khodiguian N, et al. Exercise in gestational diabetes. An optional therapeutic approach? Diabetes. 1991;40(Suppl 2):182-5.
16. Oken EY, Ning SL, Rifas-ShimanJS, et al. Association of physical activity and inactivity before and during pregnancy with glucose tolerance. Obst Gyncol. 2006 408(5): 1200-7.

17. McMurray RG, Mottola MF, Wolfe LA, et al. Recent advances in understanding maternal and fetal responses to exercise. Med Sci Sports Exerc. 1993;25:1305-21.
18. Persinger R, Foster C, Gibson M, et al. Consistency of the talk test for exercise prescription. Med Sci Sports Exerc. 2004;36:1632-6.
19. O'Toole ML, Sawicki MA, Artal R. Structured diet and physical activity prevent postpartum weight retention. J Womens Health (Larchmt) 2003;12:991-8. [PubMed] [Full Text].
20. Cary GB, Quinn TJ. Exercise and lactation: are they compatible? Can J Appl Physiol. 2001;26:55-75.

CHAPTER 11

Insulin Therapy in Pregnancy: Initiation, Titration, and Safety Update

Rajeev Chawla, Shalini Jaggi

INTRODUCTION

Diabetes, once considered a contraindication for pregnancy, is increasingly becoming a common facet in the management of a diabetic woman. Hyperglycemia in pregnancy is associated with several maternal and fetal complications, such as macrosomia, birth trauma, cesarean section, and hypocalcemia, hypoglycemia, and hyperbilirubinemia in newborns. Thus, appropriate management of diabetes in pregnancy is essential to improve not only the maternal and fetal outcomes but also to prevent future diabetes in the infant at risk born to a diabetic mother.[1-4] As of now, no oral antidiabetic drug is considered safe in pregnancy and the American Diabetes Association-European Association for the Study of Diabetes (ADA-EASD) 2017 guidelines clearly advocate use of insulin therapy as the gold standard for use in hyperglycemia management in pregnancy besides lifestyle modification and medical nutrition therapy (MNT).

PATHOPHYSIOLOGY

Pregnancy is characterized by progressive insulin resistance that starts near midpregnancy and progresses through the third trimester as a result of increased placental hormones which have an established diabetogenic action. It is important to note that this insulin resistance rapidly decreases postdelivery, again suggesting a major contribution of these placental hormones in its pathogenesis. The cumulative effects of maternal adiposity and placental influences result in abnormalities in insulin signaling pathways, which lead to decreased glucose uptake and an increase in insulin resistance. The placenta produces human chorionic somatomammotropin (HCS) or the human placental lactogen (HPL), which stimulates pancreatic secretion of insulin in the fetus and inhibits peripheral uptake of glucose in the mother.

With the progression of pregnancy, the placenta increases in size with increase in these above mentioned hormones, resulting in an increasing insulin-resistant milieu. In a nondiabetic pregnant woman, the first- and

Table 11.1: Glycemic targets in pregnancy.

	Fasting (mg/dL)	*1 hour (mg/dL)*	*2 hour (mg/dL)*
ADA	≤95	≤140	≤120
DIPSI*	≤90	-	≤120

*DIPSI uses plasma glucose.
(ADA: American Diabetes Association; DIPSI: Diabetes in Pregnancy Study Group of India)

second-phase insulin secretory responses increase proportionately to compensate for this reduced insulin sensitivity, and this is associated with both β-cell hypertrophy and hyperplasia. However, in a woman with pregestational diabetes, this compensation may not be adequate, leading to deterioration in glycemic control while in a nondiabetic woman with an increased risk of diabetes it may lead to development of gestational diabetes.[2,3]

MONITORING OF GLYCEMIC CONTROL

Regular monitoring of blood glucose is essential for achieving optimal glycemic control and successful pregnancy outcomes in a hyperglycemic pregnancy.

- In women with preexisting diabetes, prepregnancy counseling is essential to maintain blood glucose levels (Table 11.1) and hemoglobin A1c (HbA1c) level at an acceptable level (HbA1c < 7%, ideal < 6%) prior to conception to avoid maternal and fetal complications.
- Diabetic women already on treatment need to intensively monitor their glucose levels from the beginning of conception all through their pregnancy. This should be done by self-monitoring of blood glucose (SMBG).
- Ideally a 7-point testing is recommended (fasting, prelunch, and predinner, as well as all 3 postmeal readings and bedtime or 3 am).
- In high-risk pregnancies, the frequency of monitoring may be intensified with SMBG as per the requirement.
- Continuous glucose monitoring devices are available and these devices may be useful in high-risk pregnancies to know the glycemic fluctuations and to plan proper insulin dosage.

Glycosylated Hemoglobin

Hemoglobin A1c levels have shown a consistent association with mean plasma glucose throughout pregnancy. The level of HbA1c is lower in nondiabetic pregnant women due to rapid physiological increase in red cell turnover in pregnancy. Various physiological changes in the pregnancy such as volume expansion and change in the life span of the erythrocytes cause a fall in HbA1c level during second trimester and a slight rise in the third trimester.

An HbA1c level of less than 6–6.5% is recommended for planning a pregnancy in women with diabetes and those with HbA1c more than 10% are advised against pregnancy. In the second and third trimester, an A1c of less than 6% is associated with lowest risk for large-for-gestational age infants and an A1c greater than 6.5% is associated with increased adverse outcomes. Hence, a target HbA1c of 6–6.5% is recommended, though a target of less than 6% is considered optimal if achieved without significant hypoglycemia. Due to the alteration in red cell kinetics and rapidly changing physiological glycemic levels, some authors suggest assessing HbA1c levels more frequently, even monthly, to monitor glycemic control during pregnancy. An alternative can be serum fructosamine assay reflecting glycemic control over preceding 2 weeks.

MANAGEMENT OF DIABETES IN PREGNANCY

Preexisting Type 1 and 2 Diabetes

Patients with preexisting diabetes require modification of their pharmacologic regimen to meet the changing metabolic demands of pregnancy. Insulin is preferred to achieve optimal glycemic control in pregnant diabetic patients. Traditionally, intermediate insulin, such as neutral protamine Hagedorn (NPH) insulin was given before breakfast and again before dinner or at bedtime (to avoid nocturnal hypoglycemia). A split/mixed regimen (NPH and regular or insulin analogs) given in the morning and evening may also be used to achieve good glycemic control in some of the patients.

Alternatively, short-acting regular insulins can be given 30 minutes before meal or rapid acting insulin analogs can be given right before meals, particularly during the first trimester, when nausea and anorexia (morning sickness) are common.

Ideally, nowadays a basal-bolus regime with three shots of prandial insulins just before the three major meals and a shot of basal insulin (detemir) or intermediate insulin (NPH) to take care of fasting glucose is recommended for intensive glucose control.

Adjusting insulin doses is simpler with SMBG four times a day because each component of the insulin regimen affects only 1 SMBG value. Hence, monitoring before meals and 2 hours after a meal is recommended in patients on intensive insulin regimen.

In some difficult to control diabetic pregnant patients or in some high-risk pregnancies, a continuous subcutaneous insulin infusion (CSII) pump may be used. Although there may be reduced rates of hypoglycemia with CSII pumps, maternal and perinatal outcomes have been comparable in women

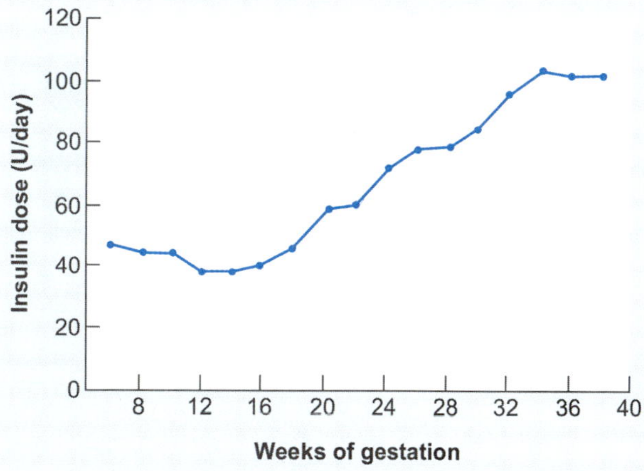

Fig. 11.1: Changing insulin requirement in a pregnant type 1 diabetic woman.

using insulin pumps versus those using multiple daily injections of regular and intermediate insulins.

In pregnant women with preexisting type 1 diabetes, insulin requirement may fall during the early part of the first trimester due to increased insulin sensitivity. However, in the later part of the pregnancy, insulin requirement increases as a result of increased levels of circulating placental hormones. Therefore, constant insulin adjustment is necessary to keep up with the increasing insulin requirement of pregnancy (Fig. 11.1). The insulin dose is increased from 0.7 U/kg/day in the first trimester to 0.8 U/kg/day at week 18, 0.9 U/kg/day at week 26, and 1.0 U/kg/day at week 36 in women who maintain within 15% of ideal body weight.

It has also been observed that pregnant women with type 2 diabetes require higher insulin dose during each trimester as compared to type 1 diabetic women. There is no difference in insulin requirement between type 1 and type 2 diabetic women during the first trimester. Subsequently, the insulin requirement significantly increases during the second trimester (10% increase for patients with type 1 diabetics as compared to 33% in those with type 2 diabetics). In the third trimester, the insulin requirement continues to rise reaching a total increment of 40% in patients with type 2 diabetes (Fig. 11.2). This can be explained due to the sudden increase in body mass and heightened insulin resistance in type 2 diabetic women during pregnancy.

It is important to remember that insulin requirement always increases during pregnancy. If this does not increase as expected, it can be a cause for concern and one should rule out poor placental growth, intrauterine growth retardation and impending intrauterine death. In some pregnant diabetics, there could be hypertrophy of fetal β-cells. These women may require less

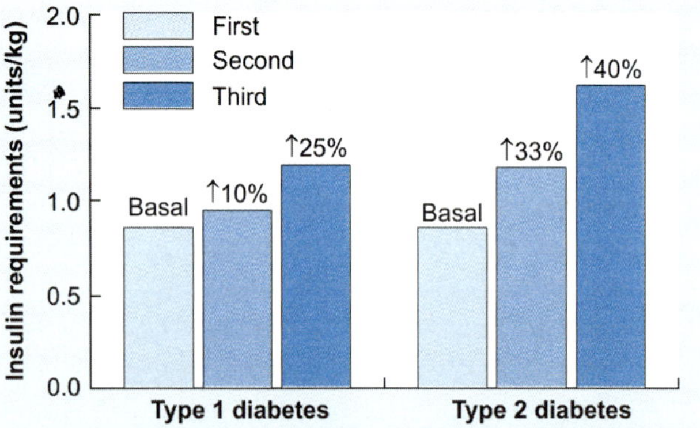

Fig. 11.2: Insulin requirement in type 1 and type 2 pregnant diabetic women.

insulin in the last week of pregnancy, which could be due to the fetal handling of maternal glucose. At approximately 36 weeks, placental growth ceases and counter regulatory hormone production plateaus. Thus, there may be an apparent decline in the insulin requirement.

Insulins

Treatment with insulin is initiated if MNT fails to achieve glycemic targets in 2 weeks in women with gestational diabetes. Insulin therapy should be individualized for each woman. NPH insulin can be started with a dose as low as 4 units and further dose can be adjusted on follow-up. Some of the patients may require combination of short-acting insulin and intermediate-acting insulin in the morning and evening.

If a patient has elevated prelunch blood glucose, regular insulin is usually necessary in the morning to handle the postbreakfast hyperglycemia, as there is a lag period before the intermediate-acting insulin begins to work. In case, postdinner blood glucose is high, a small dose of regular insulin is necessary before dinner in addition to the regular and intermediate-acting insulin given in the morning. A split-mixed dosage regimen of short- and intermediate-acting insulin in the morning and in the evening may be useful if fasting blood glucose is high. Very often, when both the premeal and postmeal sugars are elevated, a basal-bolus regime may be used for optimal glycemic control.

Insulin Analogs in Pregnancy[5]

Compared to regular insulin, the rapid acting insulin analogs are useful in diabetic pregnancies, as they are able to reduce postprandial hyperglycemia more efficiently due to their faster action. It has also been emphasized that postprandial hyperglycemia is more predictive of adverse neonatal outcomes than fasting glycemia.

All the three rapid-acting insulin analogs available in the market are more effective for early postprandial glucose control, reducing the risk of late postprandial hypoglycemia. Lispro and aspart are assigned the pregnancy category "B". Just like human regular insulin, both lispro and aspart have demonstrated clinical effectiveness, no evidence of teratogenesis, low antigenicity and placental transport of autoantibodies. Premixed insulin analogs may be considered over premixed human insulins in pregnant women for better glycemic control with lower doses of insulin and greater flexibility in the meal time insulin dosing without disturbing their routine life pattern. The doses of premixed insulins need to be adjusted during pregnancy for very tight glycemic control.

As of now, among long-acting insulins, insulin glargine has been assigned a pregnancy category "C". The current data on glargine in pregnancy shows similar fetal outcomes compared with human insulins in terms of congenital malformations. Hence, the apparent safety of glargine in pregnancy justifies the need for a large randomized controlled trial to confirm its safety and efficacy in pregnancy. On the other hand, the analog insulin detemir in pregnancy has been shifted to category "B" and can be safely used. Also currently there is no data for use of the newer insulin degludec in pregnancy as yet and hence, this insulin is not yet recommended for use in pregnancy.

Delivery Planning and Management of Diabetes during Labor

Prolongation of gestation past 39 weeks increases risk of fetal macrosomia without reducing cesarean rates; hence, delivery after 38 + 6 weeks is recommended unless obstetric considerations dictate otherwise.

In poorly controlled diabetic patients, an early elective delivery and induction of labor may be considered. Women on MNT with well-controlled diabetes and normal antenatal testing should be allowed to progress to their expected date of delivery (EDD).

Expectant management beyond the estimated due date or 40 weeks in complication free diabetic pregnancy is not recommended.

Diabetes is not an indication for cesarean section but cesarean section should be considered if fetal weight is more than 4,500 g or for any other indication such as malpresentation, disproportion, or preeclampsia.

Management for Planned Lower Segment Cesarean Section[6]

- Plan the procedure early morning.
- Give usual night dose of intermediate-acting/basal insulin.

- Nil per oral in morning—withhold morning dose of insulin.
- If surgery delayed—start corrective regimen [dextrose normal saline (DNS) with short-acting insulin, if needed] to avoid ketosis.
- Monitor blood glucose q 1-2 hourly.
- Avoid hyperglycemia during the surgery to reduce risk of neonatal hypoglycemia and wound infections in the mother.
- Intrapartum targets—maintain blood glucose between 4 mmol/L and 7 mmol/L (72-126 mg/dL).
- Maternal blood glucose value of >180 mg/dL—conclusively associated with high risk of neonatal hypoglycemia.
- Insulin requirements significantly reduce during active labor.
- Consider intravenous dextrose and insulin for women whose blood glucose is not maintained at 72-126 mg/dL. Depending on the glycemic status, insulin infusion can be started at rate of 0.5-1 U/hr. Glucose containing fluid (5% dextrose/DNS) can be started at rate of 80-125 mL/hr, either simultaneously with insulin infusion or as and when blood glucose levels <70 mg/dL. If infusion facilities are not available, subcutaneous short-acting insulin every 4-6 hourly may be given.
- Those on subcutaneous insulin infusion pumps may continue their basal infusion during labor.
- Frequent monitoring of capillary glucose is recommended due to rapid changes in glucose and consequent insulin requirement in labor:
  - q 2-4 hours during the latent phase
  - q 1-2 hours during the active phase
  - 1 hourly in patients on glucose infusion.
- For gestational diabetes mellitus (GDM) controlled only on MNT monitoring q 4-6 hour is sufficient.

Following delivery, there is a sharp fall in insulin requirement and it is advisable to decrease the insulin dose by 25-40% of the predelivery dose to prevent hypoglycemia in women with preexisting diabetes. Before discharging the patient, insulin dose should be reduced to prepregnancy levels in those with preexisting diabetes.

The newborns of diabetic mothers should also be screened and monitored for hypoglycemia, hypocalcemia, and hyperbilirubinemia. Glucose levels may remit to normal in women with GDM and insulin may be stopped in such cases based on their postpartum capillary glucose levels. 15% of GDM remain glucose intolerant or develop type 2 diabetes mellitus (T2DM) in the postpartum period and 10-50% of the women develop diabetes within 5 years of delivery.

CONCLUSION

Hyperglycemia is associated with a myriad of fetal and maternal complications in pregnancy. Various physiological mechanisms of pregnancy can result in deterioration of glycemic control in women with preexisting diabetes as well as development of gestational diabetes in women at high risk. Hence, optimal glycemic control should be achieved before planning pregnancy as well as maintained all through pregnancy. Besides lifestyle management and MNT, insulin is the treatment of choice for management of hyperglycemia in pregnancy in the absence of sufficient long-term safety data on use of other oral antidiabetic agents. None of the currently available insulins have been shown to cross placenta. Therapy should be individualized based on the type of diabetes, pattern of dysglycemia, and the targets of glycemic control in pregnancy based on frequent daily self-monitoring of blood glucose.

KEY POINTS

- Pregnancy is characterized by progressive insulin resistance that starts near midpregnancy and progresses through the third trimester and then rapidly decreases postdelivery, suggesting a major contribution of placental hormones in worsening glycemia.
- An intensive control of blood glucose levels reduces adverse maternal and fetal outcomes of hyperglycemia in pregnancy.
- Optimal glycemic control should be achieved before planning pregnancy as well as maintained all through pregnancy.
- Besides lifestyle modification and MNT, insulin is the currently recommended treatment for hyperglycemia management in the absence of convincing large scale long-term safety data on oral agent use in pregnancy.
- Insulin therapy should be individualized based on the type of diabetes, pattern of dysglycemia, and the targets of glycemic control in pregnancy based on frequent daily self-monitoring of blood glucose.

REFERENCES

1. Balaji V, Seshiah V. Management of diabetes in pregnancy. supplement to JAPI 2011;59:33-6.
2. Seshiah V, Sahay BK, Das AK, et al. Gestational diabetes mellitus—Indian guidelines. J Indian Med Assoc. 2009;107(11):799-802.
3. Seshiah V, Sahay BK, Das AK, et al. Diagnosis and management of gestational diabetes mellitus: Indian guidelines. In: Muruganathan A (Ed). Medicine Update 2013. New Delhi: Jaypee Brothers Medical Publishers (P) Ltd; 2013. pp. 201-4.
4. American Diabetes Association. Standards of Medical Care in Diabetes 2013. Diabetes Care. 2013;36(1):S11-66.
5. Torlone E, Di Cianni G, Mannino D, et al. Insulin analogs and pregnancy: an update. Acta Diabetol. 2009;46:163-72.
6. Paniker V, Sosale A, Agarwal S, et al. RSSDI Clinical Practice Recommendations for Management of In-hospital Hyperglycemia-2016. Int J Diabetes Dev Ctries. 2016;36 (Suppl 1):S1-21.

CHAPTER 12

Oral Antihyperglycemic Drugs in Pregnancy: A Review

Sachin K Jain, Ramesh Aggarwal, Anshuman Srivastava

INTRODUCTION

Diabetes is one of the most common metabolic disorders that complicate pregnancy. The prevalence of overt diabetes mellitus (DM) and gestational diabetes mellitus (GDM) has risen globally.[1] Approximately 90% of diabetes in pregnant women is attributed to GDM.[2] The incidence of GDM is 5% in the United States, and 3.8–17.9% in different parts of India.[3] Diabetes in pregnancy is associated with an increased incidence of undesirable outcomes, for both mother and infant, if the glycemic control during pregnancy is not adequate.[4] Glycemic control can be achieved by medications which leads to optimum results in diabetic pregnancies. Initial treatment is with diet and lifestyle modifications, but if it fails to achieve glycemic targets then treatment needs to be escalated. Insulin has been the gold standard therapy for DM and GDM.[5] However, insulin therapy can be inconvenient as it requires multiple daily injections, has a high cost, and requires refrigerator for storage, which results in poor patient compliance. There is a growing interest for the use of *oral antihyperglycemic drugs (OAHD)* in GDM and overt DM2 in pregnancy. The convenience of oral medications pertaining to easy dosage and cost has potential implications in low-resource settings, thus increasing the likelihood of their compliance. There are certain concerns about recommending OAHDs in pregnancy because of their possible risks of transplacental passage and consequent fetal complications.[6] This review will focus on the efficacy, safety, and recommendations of use of OAHDs in diabetes complicating pregnancy.

TREATMENT OF GESTATIONAL DIABETES MELLITUS BY ORAL ANTIHYPERGLYCEMIC DRUGS

For treatment of DM, lifestyle modification and medical nutrition therapy (MNT) remains the starting point of therapy and so in pregnancy also. However, in pregnancy, rapid control of blood glucose levels is required because of risk of developing various metabolic and developmental defects in fetus that include fetal anomalies, macrosomia, and even fetal demise.

Table 12.1: Glycemic targets in pregnancy.[7,8,10,11]

	NICE	*ADA*	*DIPSI*
Fasting	<5.3 mmol/L 95 mg/dL	<95 mg/dL	<90 mg/dL
1-hour postprandial	<7.8 mmol/L 140 mg/dL	<140 mg/dL	
Or 2-hour postprandial	<6.4 mmol/L 115 mg/dL	<120 mg/dL	<120 mg/dL

(NICE: National Institute for Health and Care Excellence; ADA; American Diabetes Association; DIPSI: Diabetes in Pregnancy Study Group India)

Neonatal hypoglycemia and hyperbilirubinemia can occur in the offspring. Antenatal complications can also occur like preeclampsia and spontaneous abortion. In addition, diabetes in pregnancy may increase the risk of obesity and DM2 in offspring later in life. A trial of MNT is started, but if it fails to achieve glycemic target (Table 12.1) within a week then therapy is required to be escalated.[7] Till now, insulin was the drug of choice in women with GDM.[8,9] Oral antidiabetic agents (OAHDs) have been used and are being studied whether they can also be used as an alternative to insulin therapy because of their ease of use and lower cost.

CURRENT POSITION OF ORAL ANTIHYPERGLYCEMIC DRUGS IN THE MANAGEMENT OF DIABETES IN PREGNANCY

Studying any drug for safety and efficacy in pregnancy has always been difficult due to ethical considerations. Historically, there had been a lot of concern about the use of OAHDs in pregnancy as these drugs were thought to cross the placenta. However, the hypothesis was not much proven as there was lack of adequate number of supporting studies. But recently, many randomized controlled trials (RCTs) and metaanalysis have shown that some of the OAHDs (glyburide and metformin) cross the placenta in insignificant amounts, whereas tolbutamide and chlorpropamide show significant trans-placental passage. Drugs like metformin, glyburide, and acarbose have been extensively studied and can be a good alternative to insulin therapy in pregnancy as they have substantial amount of data in support of their safety in pregnancy.[6,9] Various OAHDs are briefly discussed below.

Sulfonylureas

Sulfonylureas act by enhancing the release of insulin from the pancreatic beta cells. Early experience with first generation sulfonylureas (tolbutamide and chlorpropamide) resulted in severe hypoglycemia among neonates of mothers who took these drugs during pregnancy. These drugs therefore were contraindicated. Of all second generation sulfonylureas, glyburide has been studied most extensively and has shown most promising results. Elliot et al. demonstrated that glyburide does not cross the placenta in significant amounts.[9] A study done by Langer et al. showed that there were no detectable glyburide levels in the umbilical cord despite the achievement of therapeutic concentrations of the drug in the maternal blood.[6] Glyburide's inability to cross the placenta, despite its low-molecular weight, is attributed to its high protein-binding capacity of 99.8%. However, another possible explanation proposed that there was pumping back of the glyburide load back into the maternal system by an unidentified placental transport system.[12]

A systematic review done by Nicholson et al. in 2009 which included three RCTs on comparison of glyburide with insulin found no differences in glycemic control including fasting or 2-hour postprandial blood glucose (PPBG).[13] RCT done by Ogunyemi et al. showed significantly lower fasting blood glucose and 2-hour postprandial glucose in insulin group as compared to glyburide group.[14] A prospective comparative study from India done in 2013, which compared 32 patients each in glyburide and insulin group has found no significant difference in glycemic control.[15] A recent meta-analysis done by Song et al. involving 1,194 participants found no difference in maternal short-term outcomes, but the incidence of neonatal hypoglycemia was higher in the glyburide group.[16]

Fetal Outcomes

Towner et al. found that there was no association between congenital anomalies and OAHDs. The risk in individual patients appears to be related to maternal glycemic control rather than to the mode of antidiabetic therapy during early pregnancy.[17] In a meta-analysis (10 studies on 471 exposed women to sulfonylureas and biguanides in first trimester), no significant difference was found in the rate of major malformations or neonatal death among women with first trimester exposure to oral antidiabetic agents compared with nonexposed women.[18]

Study by Langer et al. showed infants born to mother with uncontrolled blood glucose levels, 17% in the glyburide group were large for gestational age, as were 19% in the insulin group; the incidence of macrosomia was 11% and 10%, respectively.[6] Among the infants of the women with adequately controlled blood glucose levels, 7% in the glyburide group and 10% in the insulin group were large for gestational age; the incidence of macrosomia was 4% and 3%, respectively highlighting the importance of good control.[6]

Maternal Outcomes

Langer et al. showed the rate of maternal hypoglycemia in the women who received insulin was higher (20%) as compared to glyburide (4%).[6] However, another study by Bertini et al., it was found to be similar.[19] In meta-analysis of three RCTs including one from India, there were similar rate of cesarean delivery, with a range between 23% and 52%.[14] Overall, maternal outcomes were similar in women treated with glyburide compared with insulin in these studies.

Biguanides

Metformin is a biguanide that functions by decreasing hepatic glucose output by inhibition of gluconeogenesis and enhanced peripheral glucose uptake. It also decreases intestinal glucose absorption and increases insulin sensitivity.[20]

Maternal Outcomes

Study done by Rowan et al. suggests that metformin is an effective and safe treatment option for women and it is more acceptable to women with GDM than is insulin.[21] Meta-analysis of three RCTs by Gui et al. comprising GDM patients showed no significant difference in average fasting and postprandial blood glucose (PPBG) levels in the metformin or the insulin group. Also there was no significant difference between the two groups in average hemoglobin A1c (HbA1c) percent level at gestational 36–37 weeks. However, metformin failure was reported in up to 46.3% patients in one of these studies.[22] The average weight gain and pregnancy-induced hypertension rates in women after enrolment was significantly higher in the insulin group than in metformin group. In the same study, there was no significant difference in the preeclampsia rate between the two groups. Average gestational ages at delivery was significantly lower in the metformin group and preterm birth rate was significantly more in the metformin group. There was no significant difference in the cesarean delivery rate between the two groups.[22]

Fetal Outcomes

Metformin has been shown to pass freely across the placenta. Two in vivo studies showed that the fetus is exposed to concentrations as high as or even higher than those seen in the mother. The studies measured maternal and cord blood samples in women taking metformin throughout pregnancy (850 mg twice daily in 15 women and 2,000 mg/day in 8 women).[23,24]

Nonrandomized studies from two groups of women during pregnancy: (1) pregnant women with polycystic ovary syndrome and (2) pregnant women with diabetes, both pregestational and gestational diabetes showed that the development of congenital anomalies that did occur in these studies was attributed to the presence of hyperglycemia during organogenesis rather than metformin. Therefore, metformin is not considered teratogenic.[20]

Gui et al. showed the average birth weight of neonates was slightly higher in the insulin group as compared with the metformin group, but the difference was not statistically significant. When compared with insulin group, the pooled result showed no significant difference between the metformin and insulin groups in large for gestational age infants rate; the small for gestational age; hypoglycemia rate; in the incidence of shoulder dystocia; neonatal intensive care unit admission; respiratory distress syndrome; hyperbilirubinemia; in-birth defect rate; birth injury rate; phototherapy rate; and in the 5-minute Apgar score.[22]

Currently an RCT known as MiTy (metformin in women with type 2 diabetes in pregnancy) trial is studying 500 women with type 2 diabetes in pregnancy to receive metformin or placebo in addition to their usual regimen of insulin (ClinicalTrials.gov). The primary outcome is a composite fetal outcome. It is in phase 3 state and the results are expected in June 2018. This study will clarify whether adding metformin to insulin in women with type 2 diabetes will be beneficial to the mothers and infants.

Alpha-glucosidase Inhibitors

Acarbose is an alpha-glucosidase inhibitor that acts at the gastrointestinal tract and delays the absorption of carbohydrates. As it is not absorbed systemically so there is no bloodstream transfer to the placenta.[11] Bertini et al. compared neonatal outcome in GDM treated with insulin, glyburide, and acarbose. They found no statistical difference in fasting and PPBG levels or average newborn weight in three groups.[19] Acarbose was found to be safe and effective oral drug and can be considered as potential oral antidiabetic drug (OAHD) for treatment of GDM.

Thiazolidinediones (Pioglitazone and Rosiglitazone)

These drugs cross the placenta and, apart from a few case studies, there is little known about their safety and efficacy in pregnancy. Study done by Chan et al. with rosiglitazone given to pregnant women undergoing surgical termination of pregnancy between 8 weeks and 12 weeks, rosiglitazone was detected in 19 out of 31 (61%) fetal samples. These drugs therefore cannot be recommended at present in pregnant diabetic women.[25]

Incretin-based Therapy

There are no human data available for recent OAHDs like dipeptidyl peptidase-4 (DPP4) inhibitors (saxagliptin, vildagliptin, and linagliptin) and oral glucagon-like peptide-1 (GLP1) analogs (semaglutide). Only one DPP4 inhibitor, sitagliptin has been studied to a limited extent and is considered as category B drug, but is not recommended for use in pregnancy.[26] Semaglutide is recently approved for use in DM2 but no studies in pregnant women are available.

CONCLUSION

Insulin is the first-line drug recommended for treatment of GDM by American Diabetes Association (ADA).[7] While individual RCTs support the efficacy and short-term safety of metformin and glyburide for the treatment of GDM, both agents cross the placenta in variable extents, long-term safety data are not yet available for any oral agent. The Endocrine Society (USA) has suggested that glyburide is suitable alternative to insulin therapy for glycemic control in women with gestational diabetes who fail to achieve sufficient glycemic control after a 1-week-trial of MNT and lifestyle modification. However, for the women with a diagnosis of GDM before 25 weeks gestation and for those women with fasting plasma glucose more than 110 mg/dL (6.1 mmol/L), insulin is the preferred therapy.[4] Starting dose of glyburide is 2.5 mg once daily and can be increased up to a maximum of 20 mg/day. The usual starting dose of metformin is 500–1,000 mg/day, which can be increased gradually up to a maximum dose of 2,500 mg/day. The use of OAHDs in pregnancies is recommended with caution by the ADA, whereas UK National Institute for Health and Care Excellence (NICE) guidelines considers metformin and glyburide safe in pregnancy and lactation. In Scotland, the Scottish Intercollegiate Guidelines Network (SIGN publication no. 116; 2010) suggested that metformin or glyburide may be considered as initial pharmacological, glucose lowering treatment in women with gestational diabetes.[27] No OAD is approved by the US Food and Drug administration (FDA) for treatment of diabetes in pregnancy.[7,8] National guidelines for the management of GDM 2014 (Government of India)[28] does not approve the use of OAHDs. We suggest that glyburide and metformin either individually or in combination may be started in women where mild GDM is detected after 25 weeks gestation and in those who are not likely to use insulin due to unavailability or reluctance in using insulin. However, more studies are needed to establish the long-term safety of OAHDs for their use in patients with GDM and overt DM2.

REFERENCES

1. Jovanovic L, Pettitt DJ. Gestational diabetes mellitus. JAMA. 2001;286(20):2516-8.
2. Guariguata L, Linnenkamp U, Beagley J, et al. Global estimates of the prevalence of hyperglycaemia in pregnancy. Diabetes Res Clin Pract. 2014;103:176-85.
3. Mithal A, Bansal B, Kalra S. Gestational diabetes in India: Science and society. Indian J Endocrinol Metab. 2015;19(6):701-4.
4. Blumer I, Hadar E, Hadden DR, et al. Diabetes and pregnancy: An endocrine society clinical practice guideline. J Clin Endocrinol Metab. 2013;98:4227-49.
5. American College of Obstetricians and Gynecologists Committee on Practice Bulletins—Obstetrics. ACOG Practice Bulletin. Clinical management guidelines for obstetrician-gynecologists. Number 30, September 2001 (replaces Technical Bulletin Number 200, December 1994). Gestational diabetes. Obstet Gynecol. 2001;98:525-38.
6. Langer O, Conway DL, Berkus MD, et al. A comparison of glyburide and insulin in women with gestational diabetes mellitus. N Engl J Med. 2000;343(16):1134-8.

7. American Diabetes Association. Standards of medical care in diabetes—2016: Summary of Revisions. Diabetes Care. 2016;39 (Suppl 1):S4-5.
8. NICE. (2015). Diabetes in pregnancy: management of diabetes and its complications from preconception to the postnatal period. [online] Available from: https://www.nice.org.uk/guidance/ng3 [Acessed December 2017].
9. Elliot B, Langer O, Schenker S, et al. Insignificant transfer of glyburide occurs across the human placenta. Am J Obstet Gynecol. 1991;165:807-12.
10. Metzger BE, Gabbe SG, Persson B, et al. International Association of Diabetes and Pregnancy Study Groups Consensus Panel, International association of diabetes and pregnancy study groups recommendations on the diagnosis and classification of hyperglycemia in pregnancy. Diabetes Care. 2010;33:676-82.
11. Seshiah V, Das AK, Balaji V, et al. Gestational diabetes mellitus—Guidelines for Diabetes In Pregnancy Study Group (DIPSI). J Assoc Physicians India. 2006;54:622-8.
12. Kalra B, Gupta Y, Singla R, et al. Use of oral anti-diabetic agents in pregnancy: A pragmatic approach. N Am J Med Sci. 2015;7(1):6-12.
13. Nicholson W, Bolen S, Witkop CT, et al. Benefits and risks of oral diabetes agents compared with insulin in women with gestational diabetes: A systematic review. Obstet Gynecol. 2009;113:193-205.
14. Ogunyemi D, Jesse M, Davidson M. Comparison of glyburide versus insulin in management of gestational diabetes mellitus. Endocr Pract. 2007;13:427-8.
15. Tempe A, Mayanglambam RD. Glyburide as treatment option for gestational diabetes mellitus. J Obstet Gynaecol Res. 2013;39:1147-52.
16. Song R, Chen L, Chen Y, et al. Comparison of glyburide and insulin in the management of gestational diabetes: A meta-analysis. PLoS One. 2017;12(8):e0182488.
17. Towner D, Kjos SL, Leung B, et al. Congenital malformations in pregnancies complicated by NIDDM. Diabetes Care. 1995;18:1446-51.
18. Gutzin SJ, Kozer E, Magee LA, et al. The safety of oral hypoglycemic agents in the first trimester of pregnancy: A meta-analysis. Can J Clin Pharmacol. 2003;10:179-83.
19. Bertini AM, Silva JC, Taborda W, et al. Perinatal outcomes and the use of oral hypoglycemic agents. J Perinat Med. 2005;33:519-23.
20. Refuerzo JS. Oral hypoglycemic agents in pregnancy. Obstet Gynecol Clin North Am. 2011;38:227-34.
21. Rowan JA, Haugue WM, Gao W, et al. Metformin versus insulin for the treatment of gestational diabetes. N Engl J Med. 2008;358:2003-15.
22. Gui J, Liu Q, Feng L. Metformin vs insulin in the management of gestational diabetes: A meta-analysis. PLoS One. 2013;8:e64585.
23. Vanky E, Zahlsen K, Spigset O, et al. Placental passage of metformin in women with polycystic ovary syndrome. Fertil Steril. 2005;83:1575-8.
24. Charles B, Norris R, Xiao X, et al. Population pharmacokinetics of metformin in late pregnancy. Ther Drug Monit. 2006;28:67-72.
25. Chan LY, Yeung JH, Lau TK. Placental transfer of rosiglitazone in the first trimester of human pregnancy. Fertil Steril. 2005;83(4):955-8.
26. Seshadri KG, Kirubha MHB. Gliptins: A new class of oral antidiabetic agents. Indian J Pharm Sci. 2009;71(6):608-14.
27. Scottish Intercollegiate Guidelines Network. (2014). Management of diabetes: A national clinical guideline. [online] Available from: http://www.sign.ac.uk/assets/sign116.pdf [Accessed December 2017].
28. National health mission. (2014) National Guidelines for Diagnosis & Management of Gestational Diabetes Mellitus. [online] Available from: http://nhm.gov.in/nrhm-components/rmnch-a/maternal-health/guidelines.html [Accessed December 2017].

CHAPTER 13

Pregnancy in a Woman with Diabetic Nephropathy

Narinder Pal Singh, Anish Kumar

INTRODUCTION

The incidence and prevalence of diabetes throughout the world are rising, leading to an increase in the incidence and prevalence of diabetic nephropathy. Currently, more than 50% of patients with end-stage renal disease (ESRD) have diabetes. Although diabetes is less common among women of child-bearing age, the number of women entering pregnancy with diabetes is rising and developing kidney disease. It is usually due to classic diabetic nephropathy, which is characterized by albuminuria and progressive chronic kidney disease (CKD; i.e. proteinuria, hematuria or decreased glomerular filtration rate (GFR) for 3 or more months, irrespective of cause).

In women with diabetic kidney disease who become pregnant, the presence of kidney disease raises important questions about the effects of the kidney disease on pregnancy outcome and the effects of pregnancy on risk of progressive kidney dysfunction. Women with pregestational diabetes, with or without nephropathy, have a higher risk of adverse pregnancy outcomes than nondiabetic women. Although it has been suggested that pregnancy negatively affects renal function in women with pregestational diabetes, pregnancy itself does not appear to adversely affect the progression of kidney disease if kidney function is normal or near normal at the start of pregnancy.

Diabetes mellitus during pregnancy may also subsequently affect metabolism and renal function in the off spring. It is speculated that abnormal in utero exposure in the off spring of diabetic mothers leads to impaired nephrogenesis and reduced nephron mass, and putting the offspring at higher risk for development of renal disease and hypertension in later life. The management and outcome of pregnancy complicated by diabetic kidney disease will be reviewed here.

EFFECT OF PREGNANCY ON DIABETIC KIDNEY DISEASE

Albuminuria

Categories of albuminuria and proteinuria in nonpregnant adults have been defined by Kidney Disease Improving Global Outcomes (KDIGO).[1]

Table 13.1: Normal laboratory values for creatinine and proteinuria in pregnancy.

	Nonpregnant	*First trimester (1–12 weeks)*	*Second trimester (12–28 weeks)*	*Third trimester (28+ weeks)*
Creatinine (μmol/L)	65–101	52–68	44–64	55–73
24-hour creatinine clearance mL/min	70–140	140–162	139–169	119–139
24-hour protein (g)	<0.15	<0.3	<0.3	<0.3

Source: Adapted from Nelson Piercy C et al.; 2010.[4]

Normal pregnancy is associated with an up to 60% increase in GFR accompanied by a modest decline in serum creatinine, and an increase in albuminuria excretion rate (Table 13.1). This increase in proteinuria is likely secondary to maladaptation to gestational changes in hyperfiltration, antiangiogenic factors, and cessation of renin-angiotensin-aldosterone system (RAAS) blockade. In women with diabetic kidney disease, albuminuria also typically increases as pregnancy progresses, and regresses to or near prepregnancy levels after delivery.[2]

Kidney Function

In women with kidney disease (estimated GFR below 60 mL/min/1.73 m^2 or albuminuria), kidney function may decline during pregnancy. Whether pregnancy causes long-term worsening of diabetic kidney disease or hastens the progression to ESRD is controversial.

In nonpregnant patients with or without diabetes, serum creatinine above 1.5 mg/dL and hypertension are the two major risk factors for progression of CKD. During pregnancy, there is concern that women with CKD who develop decreasing GFR, worsening hypertension, and/or increasing proteinuria may be at risk of accelerated progression to ESRD.[3]

However, diabetic women with normal albumin excretion or only albuminuria with normal GFR appear to be at less risk for development or progression of kidney disease compared with those who have reduced GFR. However, permanent GFR loss or ESRD may develop in women with poorly controlled hypertension or CKD at the onset of pregnancy. It appears that some of these women require dialysis or kidney transplantation sooner than if they had not become pregnant.[2]

EFFECT OF DIABETIC KIDNEY DISEASE ON PREGNANCY

Perinatal morbidity and mortality related to diabetic kidney disease have improved significantly in parallel with efforts to achieve stringent glycemic control. Despite good glycemic control, CKD is associated with an increased risk of a variety of pregnancy complications, including fetal growth restriction, abnormal antenatal fetal assessment tests (nonreactive nonstress tests, low biophysical profile scores), and preeclampsia. As a consequence, medically or obstetrically indicated preterm delivery and cesarean birth are often required.[2]

The severity of CKD directly correlates with the risk of pregnancy complications. Women with preserved kidney function (i.e. normal serum creatinine concentration) had less preterm birth than with moderate renal impairment.

Women with diabetic nephropathy, either moderately elevated serum creatinine (> 1.5 mg/dL or proteinuria > 3 g/24 hrs), were at increased risk of preterm delivery, low birth weight, and preeclampsia.

Preeclampsia is the most frequent complication of pregnancy in women with diabetic kidney disease. The risk may be related, in part, to early pregnancy hypertension, level of kidney function, level of proteinuria, or pre-existing vascular damage.[5]

It is very difficult to make the diagnosis of preeclampsia in patients who enter pregnancy with diabetic nephropathy, including hypertension and "significant" proteinuria. Escalation of both hypertension and the quantity of protein in the urine is nearly universal in these women in the third trimester, inevitably making the diagnosis of preeclampsia somewhat arbitrary in some or many cases.[2]

However, in women with prepregnancy hypertension and CKD, it can be difficult to distinguish preeclampsia from the physiological effects of pregnancy on blood pressure and albumin or protein excretion, unless preeclampsia has severe features (e.g. thrombocytopenia and elevated liver enzymes).

MANAGEMENT PRINCIPLES

Prepregnancy Optimization

All women with diabetic nephropathy should be offered prepregnancy counseling to inform them of potential adverse outcomes, enable them the opportunity to optimize glycemic and hypertension control, and to improve pregnancy outcomes. Ideally, pregnancy will be delayed until optimum maternal medical status is achieved.

The aim of prepregnancy optimization is also to reduce proteinuria with RAAS blockade, although current guidelines are conflicting. The American Diabetes Association (ADA)[6] recommends that angiotensin converting enzyme inhibitor/angiotensin receptor blockers (ACEI/ARBs) should be stopped in any sexually active woman of childbearing potential because of the risk for congenital abnormalities. The *NICE*[7] guideline for the management of diabetes in pregnancy recommend continuation of RAAS blockade until conception to minimize the length of time that women with diabetic nephropathy are suboptimally treated while trying to conceive.

Women who are not preparing for pregnancy are advised to take contraception. Estrogen-containing preparations usually are contraindicated in women with diabetic nephropathy because of an increased risk for thrombosis, cardiovascular disease, and the progression of albuminuria. Progesterone-only preparations, including oral contraceptives and implantable and intrauterine devices, are preferred. Prepregnancy optimization[8] is summarized in Table 13.2.

Table 13.2: Prepregnancy optimization and antenatal management.
Prepregnancy:
• Laboratory investigations at baseline (preferably prepregnancy): – Full blood count – Urea, creatinine, electrolytes, and uric acid – Liver function tests, albumin, and coagulation profile – HbA1C – Albumin creatinine ratio (ACR) or protein creatinine ratio (PCR) – 24-hour urine collection for quantification of proteinuria • Assessment of glycemic control: – Multidisciplinary team advice and monitoring – Target blood glucose 60–100 mg/dL (3.5–5.9 mmol) – Aim for prepregnancy HbA1c 6.5% – Dietary review with weight loss if necessary intensive treatment of hypertension and proteinuria – Maximize RAAS blockade then stop at conception – Regular pregnancy testing • Start folic acid 5 mg once daily (prepregnancy) until 12 weeks • Smoking cessation • Microvascular risk assessment: – Retinopathy assessment – ECG with or without 2D echocardiogram • Ensure reliable contraception method is used until optimal HbA1c and blood pressure are achieved
Antenatal care:
• Regular multidisciplinary team visits (contact every 1–2 weeks throughout gestation): – Continue intensive glycemic control – Target blood pressure systolic 110–130 mm Hg; diastolic 70–90 mm Hg – At least 4 weekly serum creatinine and ACR checks and at least 2 weekly starting from 32 weeks gestation – Retinopathy assessment in first trimester if not done within 3 months before conception, repeat again at 28 weeks if normal or at 16–20 weeks if retinopathy is present

Contd...

Contd...

• Medication changes: – Start aspirin 75–81 mg once daily (continue prepregnancy or at confirmation of conception) – Stop RAAS blockade and other antihypertensives and statin – Start pregnancy safe antihypertensives, e.g. nifedipine and methyldopa – Switch to insulin if type 2 diabetes – Treat vitamin D deficiency if present (e.g. cholecalciferol 20,000 IU every 2 weeks until replete) – Consider thromboprophylaxis if there is high risk for thrombosis • Fetal monitoring – Nuchal scan at 11–13 weeks – Fetal cardiac scan, four-chamber view and outflow tracts at 18–20 weeks – Uterine artery Doppler at 20–24 weeks – Regular fetal monitoring to detect growth restriction or macrosomia every 4 weeks from 28 weeks to 36 weeks • Offer induction of labor or cesarean section if indicated at 37–38 weeks
Peripartum:
• Delivery in center with neonatal support • Type 1 diabetes, intravenous insulin during labor
Postpartum:
• Neonatal monitoring for hypoglycemia • Restart RAAS blockade as soon as renal function is stable (e.g. enalapril, captopril if breastfeeding)

(HbA1c: Hemoglobin A1c; RAAS: Renin-angiotensin-aldosterone system)
Source: Adapted from Kate Bramham et al.; 2017.[8]

MANAGEMENT DURING PREGNANCY

Antenatal care for women with diabetic nephropathy should be provided by a multidisciplinary team with experience in high-risk pregnancies who continually focus on maintaining tight glycemic and hypertension control in the mother and frequently monitor the fetus.

Glycemic Control

Neutral protamine Hagedorn (NPH) insulin remains the first-line treatment recommended by current guidelines.[9] Metformin and sulfonylureas are considered safe in pregnancy, but oral hypoglycemic agents have been shown to be inferior to insulin for achieving adequate glycemic control. Thus, women with type 2 diabetes are recommended to switch to insulin after conception.[10]

Hemoglobin A1c (HbA1c) loses accuracy for glycemic control during pregnancy because of the increased red blood cell turnover and other metabolic changes. Glycosuria is also inaccurate at monitoring diabetes during pregnancy because it is frequently present in women without diabetes due to saturation of renal tubular uptake. For this reason, most specialists do not use HbA1c for monitoring glycemic control; however, HbA1c above 6.5% recently has been demonstrated in women with type 1 diabetes to be a predictor of adverse pregnancy outcomes, including preeclampsia, preterm delivery, and large for gestational age infants.[11]

Blood Pressure Control

For pregnant women, who require antihypertensive therapy, systolic blood pressure (SBP) levels of 120–160 mm Hg and diastolic blood pressure (DBP) levels of 80–105 mm Hg are suggested to optimize maternal health without risking fetal harm. Lower targets (SBP 110–119 mm Hg and DBP 65–79 mm Hg) may contribute to improved long-term maternal health; however, they may be associated with impaired fetal growth. Pregnant women with hypertension and evidence of end-organ damage from cardiovascular and/or renal disease may be considered for lower blood pressure targets to avoid progression of these conditions during pregnancy. *Labetalol* does not appear to affect uteroplacental blood flow, and can be given orally or parenterally; however, other beta-blockers, particularly nonselective beta blockers, have been associated with lower placental and fetal weight when used early in pregnancy, myometrial relaxation, and premature labor. *Hydralazine* has a good safety profile in pregnancy, and can be given orally or parenterally, but can be associated with reflex tachycardia and fluid retention. Data on the safety of *calcium channel blockers* during pregnancy are mixed. Long-acting nifedipine has been used without major problems. Although amlodipine is widely used in nonpregnant individuals with hypertension, there are sparse data of its use in pregnancy. Use of diltiazem and verapamil, in women with albuminuria, reduce both blood pressure and proteinuria, although limited data available in pregnancy but no evidence of adverse fetal effects. *Methyldopa* has been used safely for many years, but is only modestly effective and has sedating effects. *Clonidine* has a similar mechanism of action to methyldopa. It can be given orally or as a transcutaneous patch; abrupt discontinuation should be avoided, if possible, as rebound increases in blood pressure can occur. *Thiazide diuretic* use during pregnancy is controversial; volume depletion is unusual, but patients should be monitored for potential changes in serum electrolytes. *ACEI/ARBs* are contraindicated during pregnancy because of teratogenic risk. Notably, these medications are toxic to the fetus if exposure occurs during the second or third trimester, leading to adverse outcomes, including hypocalvaria, renal tubular dysplasia, and IUGR. Although surveillance studies find little to no adverse fetal consequences among women taking ACEIs in the first trimester, exencephaly and unilateral renal agenesis were found in the fetus of a mother who was taking an ARB at conception. Therefore, although preconception and postpartum (e.g. during breastfeeding) use of these medications appears to be safe, exposure during pregnancy, especially in the second or third trimester, is contraindicated.[7]

Prevention of Preeclampsia

As discussed above, women with diabetic kidney disease are at increased risk of developing preeclampsia. Use low-dose aspirin prophylaxis for pregnant women at moderate to high risk of developing preeclampsia. A modest reduction in the risk of preeclampsia is possible; however, we believe no prophylaxis is also reasonable, given that experts have been unable to identify a group of pregnant women who will predictably derive a clinically significant benefit from low-dose aspirin therapy and there is no consensus on criteria to define women at moderate to high risk for preeclampsia.

Diagnosis of superimposed preeclampsia in women with diabetic nephropathy might be challenging due to the exacerbation of hypertension and proteinuria with gestation.

Antenatal Care

In addition to standard obstetrical care, we recommend the following in women with diabetic kidney disease:

- Although there is no universal standard for how often a patient's kidney function should be monitored, many institutions measure urine albumin-to-creatinine ratio in an untimed urinary sample at least monthly. Serum creatinine can be used to estimate GFR in individuals with stable kidney function. Intervention because of worsening kidney function (i.e. falling creatinine clearance, increasing blood pressure, development of uremia) is indicated if the intervention may have favorable maternal or fetal consequences, and should be individualized for each patient.
- Monitor blood pressure at least monthly. ACE inhibitors and ARBs should *not* be used. Home blood pressure monitoring should be encouraged. Ambulatory blood pressure monitoring may also be helpful in gauging blood pressure values, or response to therapy.
- Sonographic assessment of fetal growth every 4–6 weeks in the last half of pregnancy. Diabetic kidney disease does not influence the management of intrauterine growth restriction or macrosomia (estimated fetal weight >4,500 g), if present.
- Fetal assessment with nonstress tests or biophysical profile score or a combination of these tests twice per week is begun at 32 weeks, but may be initiated as early as 26 weeks in patients who develop obstetrical indications for fetal assessment (e.g. intrauterine growth restriction and preeclampsia).
- The role of dietary protein restriction is uncertain in individuals with diabetic nephropathy, particularly during pregnancy. It is reasonable,

however, to avoid a high-protein diet by limiting protein intake to a level at which compliance is not difficult for the patient.

COMORBIDITIES

Retinopathy

Diabetic retinopathy is common in women with diabetic nephropathy and may deteriorate in pregnancy due to improved blood glucose control and increased blood flow, particularly in those with established disease, anemia, diastolic hypertension, and type 1 diabetes; however, this should not be a contraindication to achieving target blood levels or a vaginal delivery. Laser treatment can be given for treatment or prevention of retinopathy during pregnancy.[12]

Cardiovascular Health

Women with diabetic nephropathy are at increased risk of cardiovascular disease matched for age with nondiabetic individuals. Substantial reduction in high-density lipoprotein level is recognized in pregnancy, which could exacerbate pre-existing dyslipidemia. Statins should be discontinued in pregnancy and prepregnancy due to potential teratogenicity.[13]

Thromboembolic Disease

Proteinuria is associated with hypercoagulability due to alterations in coagulation factors and loss of antithrombin in the urine. This, coupled with the sixfold increase in venous thromboembolic events (VTEs) reported in pregnancy, suggests that women with heavy proteinuria in pregnancy might be anticipated to be at high risk of VTE. British guidelines suggest that any woman with proteinuria of above 2 g/24 hrs and serum albumin below 20 g/L should receive thromboprophylaxis throughout pregnancy and 6 weeks postpartum, but risk should be regularly assessed in the light of additional factors, e.g. hospital admission, concurrent infection, dehydration, preeclampsia, etc.[14]

RENAL REPLACEMENT THERAPY IN PREGNANCY

In view of poor pregnancy outcomes in women with deteriorating renal function, renal replacement therapy is recommended. Hemodialysis is currently the treatment of choice. Erythropoietin production increases several fold in pregnancy and erythropoiesis-stimulating agent (ESAs) may be required in women with more severe disease. Table 13.3 provides recommendations for managing hemodialysis during pregnancy. Other management principles which are necessary for a successful pregnancy outcome include:[15]

- Control of maternal BP, generally to 110 to 140/80 to 90 mm Hg. This is difficult to achieve in many women. First, despite little or no endogenous renal function, there still appears to be volume expansion in women on maintenance hemodialysis who become pregnant, as evidenced by anemia and fall in serum albumin. To date, no data recommend assessing volume status in dialysis patients during pregnancy by measurements such as ultrasound of inferior vena cava diameter or bioimpedance.
- Active management of anemia with iron and ESAs. Target hemoglobin value should be 10–11 g/dL.
- Detection and early treatment of sepsis, which may precipitate premature labor or premature rupture of membranes.

Table 13.3: Management of the pregnant dialysis patient.

Prepregnancy:	
• Discuss risks of pregnancy (miscarriage, fetal death, fetal growth restriction, prematurity, and preeclampsia). • Ensure all medications safe in pregnancy. • Aspirin: 75–150 mg daily • Folic acid: 5 mg daily	
During pregnancy:	
Dialysis	• 20 hrs/week in four or more sessions • Aim for predialysis BUN >40 mg/dL (serum urea 15 mmol/L) • Heparin requirement may increase because of hypercoagulability of pregnancy
Anemia	• Intravenous iron to maintain iron stores • Dose of erythropoiesis-stimulating agent to achieve hemoglobin of 10–11 g/dL
Bicarbonate	• Adjust oral and dialysate bicarbonate to achieve normal serum bicarbonate for pregnancy (18–22 mmol/L)
Nutrition	• Dietician advice to ensure adequate protein and nutrient intake • Supplement oral or dialysate phosphate to maintain postdialysis serum phosphate in normal range
Calcium	• Maintain normal serum calcium with additional oral calcium and vitamin D, as well as increased dialysate calcium • Hypercalcemia occasionally provoked by placental parathyroid hormone-related peptide (PTHrP) and vitamin D-like substances
Phosphate	• Supplement oral or dialysate phosphate to maintain postdialysis serum phosphate in normal range
After pregnancy:	
• Return to usual dialysis schedule immediately • Readjust dry weight and antihypertensives weekly for 6 weeks	

(BUN: Blood urea nitrogen)

(*Source*: Adapted from Brown MA et al.; 2015.[15]

PREGNANCY IN RENAL TRANSPLANT PATIENT

Fertility improves after renal transplantation. Women are advised to wait at least 1 year after living-related donor transplantation and 2 years after deceased transplantation to avoid complications arising from immunotherapy and rejection. Immunosuppressive regimens may need to be adjusted prior to attempting to conceive. *Mycophenolate mofetil* and *sirolimus* are contra-indicated in pregnancy. Women should change from *mycophenolate mofetil to azathioprine* and from *sirolimus to tacrolimus or cyclosporine* if there are no contraindications to the switch. Upon delivery, it is a practice to switch the mother back to her basal immunosuppression to prevent late acute rejection and chronic allograft nephropathy (Table 13.4).[15]

Table 13.4: General management of renal transplant recipients during pregnancy.
Prepregnancy: • Discuss risks with transplant recipient and her partner • Best pregnancy outcome will occur if: – Prepregnancy serum creatinine <1 mg/dL (125 μmol/L) – Proteinuria <500 mg/day – Blood pressure <140/90 mm Hg • Aspirin (75–150 mg/day) if creatinine ≥1.5 mg/dL (130 μmol/L) *or* 0.9–1.5 mg/dL (100–130 μmol/L) and proteinuria >1 g/day • Replace all medications that are not safe in pregnancy • Eradicate UTI before pregnancy; prophylactic antibiotics indicated if there has been recurrent UTI since transplant • Stable cyclosporine or tacrolimus blood levels • Control diabetes
During pregnancy: • Visits every 2 weeks until 24 weeks' gestation (alternating between obstetrician and nephrologist), then weekly • Assess fetal growth by ultrasound at least every 4 weeks from 24 weeks' gestation • Do not adjust CNI dose during pregnancy unless there are extreme variations from stable prepregnancy levels • Screen for gestational diabetes at 28 weeks' gestation with 1-hour 50-g glucose challenge test • At each visit, assess BP (goal 110 to 140/80 to 90 mm Hg), proteinuria (dipstick, then PC ratio if dipstick result is positive), urine culture (if history of recurrent UTI, otherwise at 24, 28, and 32 weeks of gestation), electrolytes, creatinine, full blood count, CNI level, and fetal growth. • Reassess at each visit whether there is an impending indication for delivery
During delivery: • Vaginal delivery is usually possible despite pelvic kidney • Prophylactic antibiotics are not required routinely

Contd...

Contd...

Postpartum:
• Monitor CNI and serum creatinine levels daily in hospital • Breastfeeding appears safe with CNI drugs, azathioprine, and corticosteroids, but discuss individual case with neonatologist • Review weekly or every other week for the first 3 months

(UTI: Urinary tract infection; CNI: Calcineurin inhibitor; PC Ratio: protein-creatinine ratio)
Source: Adapted from Brown MA et al.; 2015.[15]

KEY POINTS

- In women with diabetic kidney disease, albuminuria typically increases as pregnancy progresses, and regresses to or near prepregnancy levels after delivery.
- Pregnant women with diabetes and normal albumin excretion are at low risk for development of kidney disease. Pregnant women with diabetes, microalbuminuria, and normal kidney function appear to be at low risk for loss of kidney function, but may have a transient increase in albuminuria. However, women with poorly controlled hypertension or reduced GFR and increased proteinuria (serum creatinine level >1.5 mg/dL, proteinuria >3 g in 24 hours) at the onset of pregnancy are at risk of permanent kidney damage, including ESRD.
- Diabetic kidney disease is associated with an increased risk of pregnancy complications, including fetal growth restriction, abnormal antenatal fetal assessment tests (nonreactive nonstress tests, low biophysical profile scores), and preeclampsia, even in women with good glycemic control. The occurrence of these pregnancy complications may necessitate preterm delivery and increases the chance of cesarean birth.
- Pregnant women with hypertension and evidence of end-organ damage from cardiovascular and/or renal disease may be considered for lower blood pressure targets (SBP 110–119 mm Hg and DBP 65–79 mm Hg).
- Angiotensin converting enzyme inhibitor/angiotensin receptor blockers are contraindicated during all stages of pregnancy because of teratogenic risk.
- In women with chronic primary or secondary hypertension or previous pregnancy-related hypertension, low-dose aspirin from the 12th week of gestation until delivery is suggested.
- General principles of management include increased frequency of prenatal visits, early detection and treatment of asymptomatic bacteriuria, serial monitoring of maternal renal function and for the treatment of hypertension, monitoring for the development of preeclampsia and fetal surveillance with ultrasound and fetal heart rate.

- Preterm intervention may be necessitated by deteriorating renal function, severe preeclampsia, fetal growth restriction, or nonreassuring fetal testing.

REFERENCES

1. KDIGO 2012 Clinical practice guideline for the evaluation and management of the chronic kidney disease. Kidney Int. 2013;84(3):622-3.
2. Reece EA, Weir MR. 2017. Pregnancy in women with diabetic kidney disease. [online] Available from https://www.uptodate.com/contents/pregnancy-in-women-with-diabetic-kidney-disease [Accessed December 2017).
3. Biesenbach G, Grafinger P, Stöger H, et al. How pregnancy influences renal function in nephropathic type 1 diabetic women depends on their pre-conceptional creatinine clearance. J Nephrol. 1999;12(1):41-6.
4. Nelson-Piercy C (Ed). Handbook of Obstetric Medicine, 4th edition. London: Informa Healthcare; 2010.
5. Klemetti MM, Laivuori H, Tikkanen M, et al. Obstetric and perinatal outcome in type 1 diabetes patients with diabetic nephropathy during 1988-2011. Diabetologia. 2015;58(4):678-86.
6. American Diabetes Association - Standards of Medical Care in Diabetes 2017. Management of diabetes in pregnancy. Diabetes Care. 2017;40(Suppl 1):S114-19.
7. National Institute of Clinical and Health Excellence (NICE). Diabetes in pregnancy: management of diabetes and its complications from preconception to the postnatal period. NICE guideline [NG3]. 2015 [online] Available from: https://www.nice.org.uk/guidance/ng3 [Accessed December 2017].
8. Bramham K. Diabetic nephropathy and pregnancy. Semi Nephrol. 2017;37(4):362-69.
9. Pantalone KM, Faiman C, Olansky L. Insulin glargine use during pregnancy. Endocr Pract. 2011;17(3):448-55.
10. Ekpebegh CO, Coetzee EJ, van der Merwe L, et al. A 10-year retrospective analysis of pregnancy outcome in pregestational type 2 diabetes: comparison of insulin and oral glucose-lowering agents. Diabet Med. 2007;24(3):253-8.
11. Maresh MJ, Holmes VA, Patterson CC, et al; Diabetes, Pre-eclampsia Intervention Trial Study Group. Glycemic targets in the second and third trimester of pregnancy for women with type 1 diabetes. Diabetes Care. 2015;38(1):34-42.
12. Diabetes Control and Complications Trial Research Group. Effect of pregnancy on microvascular complications in the diabetes control and complications trial. Diabetes Care. 2000;23(8):1084-91.
13. Edison RJ, Muenke M. Central nervous system and limb anomalies in case reports of first-trimester statin exposure. New Engl J Med. 2004;350(15):1579-82.
14. Brown MA. Chronic kidney disease in pregnancy: patterns of care and general principles of management. In: Davison JM, Nelson-Piercy C, Kehoe S, Baker P (Eds). Renal Disease in Pregnancy, illustrated edition. London: RCOG Press; 2008. pp. 31-44.
15. Brown MA. Pregnancy with preexisting kidney disease. In: Johnson RJ, Feehally J, Floege J (Eds). Comprehensive Clinical Nephrology, 5th edition. Philadelphia, PA: Saunders, an imprint of Elsevier Inc.; 2015.

CHAPTER 14

Diabetic Retinopathy in Pregnancy

Rohan Chawla, Tarjani Makwana, Pradeep Venkatesh

INTRODUCTION

Diabetic retinopathy (DR) is the most common microvascular complication of diabetes mellitus (DM). It also accounts for the largest cause of blindness amongst middle-aged individuals in the industrialized world. Three out of four people with more than 15 years of DM develop some amount of DR. Chronic hyperglycemia is the most important risk factor leading to retinopathy and other complications of diabetes. The risk of developing DR is higher in type 1 diabetes than type 2 diabetes.[1]

Microangiopathy in patients with diabetes retinopathy results in capillary occlusion on one hand and vascular leakage causing diabetic macular edema on the other. Capillary occlusion causes retinal ischemia, which increases the level of vascular endothelial growth factor (VEGF). This is responsible for the formation of neovascularization and the proliferative stage of DR. Biochemical alterations such as oxidative stress, activation of protein kinase C, and formation of advanced glycation end products have also been detected as a response of the retina to hyperglycemia.[1] Some studies have suggested a possible role of elevated serum insulin-like growth factor-I (IGF-I) for accelerating DR during pregnancy. The effect of IGF-I is not fully understood, but interaction between IGF-I and its receptor is probably necessary for induction of neovascularization by VEGF.[2]

Pregnancy is an established risk factor for progression of retinopathy. There is a definite increased prevalence and severity of retinopathy in pregnant women as compared to nonpregnant diabetic women. Women with type I diabetes are more likely to develop ocular changes during pregnancy.[3] Progression of retinopathy in pregnancy is defined as a deterioration corresponding to at least one stage between two examinations.[4] The factors associated with progression of DR include the pregnant state itself, duration of diabetes, amount of retinopathy at conception, blood glucose control, and the presence of coexisting hypertension (Box 14.1). Although the rate of regression of DR at the end of pregnancy or the postpartum period is high, careful monitoring of these patients is necessary to prevent diminution of

Box 14.1: Factors associated with progression of diabetic retinopathy during pregnancy.

- Duration of diabetes
- Amount of retinopathy at conception
- Blood glucose control
- Presence of coexisting hypertension
- Anemia

vision and to optimize the outcome of pregnancy.[5] The Diabetes Control and Complications Trial (DCCT) Research Group and the Diabetes in Early Pregnancy (DIEP) study, both large prospective studies with 180 and 140 patients, respectively, have provided information on the effects of pregnancy on the development and progression of DR.[6,7] Some studies suggest that pregnancy may be protective, preventing the progression of DR in the long-term.[8]

Hormonal changes, changes in the systemic vasculature and retinal autoregulatory mechanisms may be responsible for the worsening of retinopathy during pregnancy. Hormonal changes in pregnancy include increase plasma levels of human placental lactogen, estrogen, and progesterone. These may induce vascular changes leading to progression of retinopathy in pregnancy.[9] The autoregulatory mechanism is impaired in DR due to the loss of capillary pericytes and this may be further worsened in pregnancy.[10] Thus, in a diabetic patient, the physiological changes of pregnancy are an additional stress factor on an already compromised retinal circulation.

Pregnancy itself does not cause any long-term detrimental effects on the retina, kidney, and peripheral nervous system. Diabetic macular edema and proliferative retinopathy can develop during pregnancy in pre-existing diabetics. The macular edema and proliferative retinopathy have a tendency to regress postpartum. However, the presence of macular edema at an early stage in pregnancy poses a significant risk for irreversible damage to the retina.[11] The adverse effect of pregnancy on the retinal microvasculature is relatively transient, with risk of progression to proliferative diabetic retinopathy (PDR) being high only within the first 8 weeks after delivery (Fig. 14.1). This increased risk may persist into the first year postpartum, but eventually diminishes.[7]

EFFECT OF DIABETIC RETINOPATHY ON PREGNANCY[12,13]

Several studies have looked into the possibility of a relation between DR and the perinatal outcome. Women with severe form of disease are more likely to develop obstetric complications compared to women with no retinal or minimal retinal changes. Incidence of congenital malformations and/or fetal death is more in patients with proliferative changes. The severity of

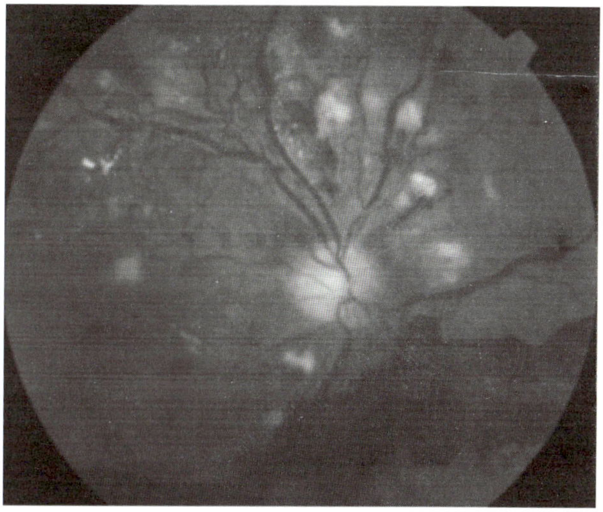

Fig. 14.1: Fundus photograph of the right eye of a patient with proliferative diabetic retinopathy. Neovascularization is noted along the superior arcade. Pre-retinal bleed is noted along the inferior arcade and inferior to the optic disk. *(for color version see Plate 3)*

retinopathy correlates with the presence of angiopathy elsewhere in the body, especially the kidneys.

MANAGEMENT OF DIABETIC RETINOPATHY DURING PREGNANCY

As DR can worsen during pregnancy, diabetic women should have preconception counseling and follow-up by a multidisciplinary team consisting of endocrinologist, ophthalmologist, gynecologist, and perinatologist. The patient should be clearly explained about the risk of progression of DR and the importance of a good metabolic control before and throughout pregnancy. Patients with a longer duration of pregnancy, severe retinopathy at baseline, coexisting hypertension, and renal disease need a closer follow-up.

The American Diabetes Association (ADA) recommends the following as optimal glycemic goals for women with pre-existing type I or type II DM planning pregnancy:[4]

- Premeal, bedtime, and overnight glucose 60–99 mg/dL
- Peak postprandial glucose 100–129 mg/dL
- Hemoglobin A1c below 6.0%
- Blood pressure less than 130/80 mm Hg during the 9 months of pregnancy.

The American Academy of Ophthalmology recommends that pregnant diabetic women should have an ophthalmological examination before conception to determine the baseline severity and then again during the first trimester. Subsequent examination should be every 3 months until delivery.[14]

Table 14.1: Recommendations for management of pregnant patients with type I diabetes mellitus to decrease the risk of progression of diabetic retinopathy (DR).

Time period	*Recommendations*
Preconception	• Counseling of diabetic women in childbearing years (especially those with pre-existing DR) about the risk of progression • Discuss postponement of conception until ocular disease is treated and stabilized • Diabetic patient should be brought under optimal glycemia control before conception • Counsel patients about benefits of early pregnancy planning • Comprehensive eye examination to detect pre-existing DR and define the baseline level
First trimester	• Comprehensive eye assessment • Frequent monitoring of blood pressure • Tight glycemic control: First diet control and if blood sugar not controlled initiate insulin therapy
Second trimester and third trimester	• Comprehensive eye examination at the discretion of the examiner but preferably every 3 months until delivery • Monitor blood pressure • Tight glycemic control
Postpartum	• Recommendations are conflicting • Some sources suggest frequent ophthalmologic surveillance for at least first year postpartum

According to the NICE guidelines, retinal assessment during pregnancy should be done by digital imaging with mydriasis using tropicamide 1% following the first antenatal clinic appointment and again at 28 weeks if the first assessment is normal. If during the first assessment, there were any DR changes the patient should be seen again around 16–20 weeks. Women with preproliferative changes during pregnancy should further have a 6 monthly follow-up after delivery.[15]

Recommendations for Management of Pregnant Patients with Type I DM to Decrease the Risk of Progression of DR[16]

Recommendations have been shown in Table 14.1.

In patients with longer duration of diabetes, every effort should be taken to achieve a good metabolic control preferably over a period of weeks or months before conception. If it is not possible, blood sugar levels should be normalized as soon as possible during pregnancy.

Patients with severe nonproliferative and proliferative changes have a greater tendency for progression during pregnancy. In such patients pregnancy, should be deferred till the eye disease is treated and stabilized. If progression of the eye disease is noted during pregnancy, prompt laser photocoagulation is indicated in eyes with severe nonproliferative changes and

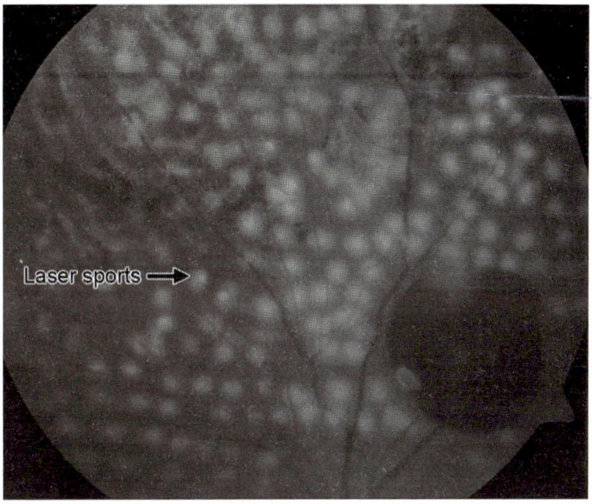

Fig. 14.2: Fundus photograph of a patient with proliferative diabetic retinopathy in which pan retinal photocoagulation has been performed. Fresh laser spots are seen (black arrow). *(for color version see Plate 3)*

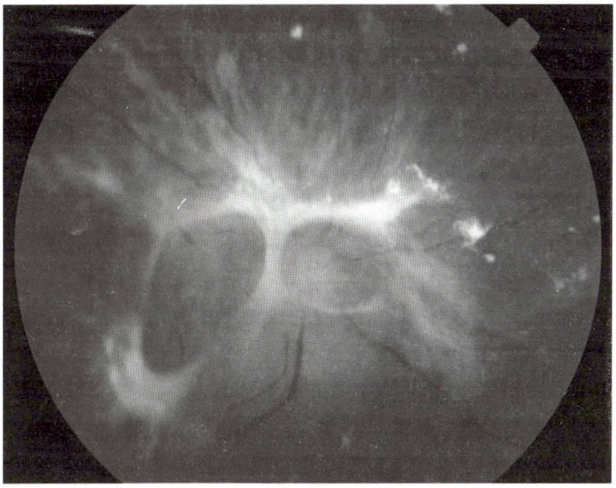

Fig. 14.3: Fundus image showing a large tractional retinal detachment extending from nasal to the optic disk toward the macula. *(for color version see Plate 3)*

should not be delayed till proliferative changes develop. Laser photocoagulation is the mainstay of treatment for DR with reasonable outcomes[17] (Fig. 14.2). Indications for surgery during pregnancy include tractional retinal detachment, nonclearing vitreous hemorrhage, and neovascular glaucoma.[18] Retinal surgery in pregnant women may be difficult, because of the potential problem of pregnant women to lie flat and prone for a considerable period of time. Moreover presence of neovascular glaucoma with tractional detachment may be associated with a poor visual outcome[18] (Fig. 14.3).

Diabetic retinopathy with proliferative changes also shows a strong tendency toward regression after delivery. Patients with severe changes should be closely followed-up in the postpartum period till the diabetic retinal changes stabilize. This includes close retinal surveillance during the first year postpartum.

If macular edema is noted during pregnancy, laser treatment might be effective. But because of high rates of regression postpartum, some studies recommend withholding laser treatment for macular edema.[19] It may be considered in severe cases or when diabetic macular edema is seen very early in pregnancy.

Intravitreal Antivascular Endothelial Growth Factor Therapy for Diabetic Retinopathy in Pregnancy

Antivascular endothelial growth factor (Anti-VEGF) therapy is now a mainstay of management of diabetic macular edema and selected cases of proliferative retinopathy in nonpregnant patients. At present, anti-VEGF use in pregnancy is not well defined and has been used only in case reports or small case series during pregnancy. Prospective studies on the effects of intravitreal anti-VEGF in pregnant women are lacking. It is known that the first trimester is crucial for the fetal development. In humans, susceptibility to teratogens is maximal during organogenesis (3–8 weeks postconception), when the tissues and organs are forming. Although the function and maturation of these organs may be affected at later stages, structural defects usually occur during these early phases of development.[20] Following an intravitreal injection of an anti-VEGF agent, the systemic levels do not rise very high. Yet until more is known about this, it seems reasonable to avoid treatment with these drugs a few weeks before and at least during the first trimester of pregnancy.[21] Even in the second and third trimester they should only be used if thought to be extremely essential for preserving vision and only after taking a proper informed consent from the patient. Most of the reports of anti-VEGF (bevacizumab in a dose 1.25 mg/0.05 mL) use during pregnancy are not from cases of DR but for other retinal disorders such as myopic choroidal neovascularization or presumed ocular histoplasmosis syndrome. Also they were given in previously unrecognized pregnancies.

In summary, progression of retinopathy in pregnancy depends on severity of retinopathy at conception, adequacy of treatment, duration of diabetes, metabolic control before pregnancy, and the presence of additional vascular damage such as pre-existing or concomitant hypertensive disorder. The risks of visual loss in patients with minimal retinopathy at the inception of pregnancy are minor, and for these mothers a fundus examination every 3 month should suffice. In those with moderate background retinopathy, fundus examination should be performed at each obstetric visit (which is usually every 4–6 weeks) and if progression is detected the patient should be examined at 2-week intervals to detect any high-risk characteristic. If severe nonproliferative diabetic retinopathy develops, photocoagulation should be carried out and monitored by fundus examination. In those with severe sight threatening retinopathy, laser photocoagulation should be performed before pregnancy or promptly after diagnosis.

In a study done at our center, the prevalence of DR was 17% in pregnant women with pre-existing type I or type II DM. Progression of DR during pregnancy was seen in 50% cases. 50% cases can have severe retinopathy (PDR) at presentation and prompt laser photocoagulation should be done in these cases. Most important risk factor was the duration of DM (14 years vs. 3.5 years) and the mean age at conception was high in patients with pre-existing DM. The numbers in our study were too small to comment on risk of abortion and fetal outcomes (though risk percentages were higher in those with retinopathy).

Patient education is an important aspect in Indian scenario. Need for completion of family early, should be stressed in these mothers. Retina evaluation before conception (Preconception screening) should also be stressed upon. Guidelines need to be developed regarding medical termination of pregnancy (MTP) vs. continuation of pregnancy in those with advanced DR at presentation.

GESTATIONAL DIABETES MELLITUS

Gestational diabetes mellitus (GDM) is defined as glucose intolerance which was not present or recognized prior to pregnancy.[22] Most commonly GDM affects 2–5% of pregnant women.[23] Insulin resistance during pregnancy might develop from a variety of factors such as alterations in growth hormone and cortisol secretion (insulin antagonists), human placental lactogen secretion (which promotes lipolysis and decreases glucose uptake), and insulinase secretion by placenta.[24]

Women who are diagnosed with gestational diabetes are not at increased risk of development of DR during pregnancy.[25]

However, there are a few reports of development of proliferative retinopathy in a gestational diabetes patient following rapid metabolic control.[26] They also found that the patients who had developed retinopathy in current pregnancy had GDM in their previous pregnancy too, but the patient had defaulted follow up after the first pregnancy.

At our center, we follow the same guidelines for screening of GDM mothers as for pregestational diabetes for retinal screening during pregnancy. Dilated fundus examination is performed once in every trimester during the course of pregnancy. Postpartum examination is not performed if the blood sugars return to normal.

CHAPTER 15

Hypertensive Disorders in Diabetic Pregnancy

Harsha Khullar

INTRODUCTION

The common conditions coexisting with type 2 diabetes are clear risk factors for atherosclerotic cardiovascular disease. Atherosclerosis and microvascular disease involving retinopathy, nephropathy, and neuropathy are the consequences of diabetes leading to increased morbidity. There has been an association between poor glycemic control and microvascular complications.

Mechanism of glycemic control predisposing to vascular disease is not clearly understood. Advanced glycation end products and sorbitol, protein kinase C, and other factors may also contribute to this mechanism.

Among women with pregestational diabetes mellitus, frequency of preeclampsia (PE) increases with increasing severity.[1] Even the insulin resistance precedes the clinical onset of hypertension in pregnancy.[2]

Prevalence of hypertension has been found to be 40.8% in type 2 diabetic pregnant women as compared to 10% in nondiabetic controls in a study by Colatrella A et al.[3]

Both spontaneous and indicated preterm deliveries are increased among women with pregestational diabetes mellitus with chronic hypertension.[4]

Organ-specific factors along with systemic factors play an important role in kidney, e.g. stimulation of mesangial matrix production by hyperglycemia, activation of protein kinase C, and an increasing degree of intraglomerular hypertension may contribute to glomerular injury.

Another important factor has been reported to be genetic.

TYPES OF HYPERTENSIVE DISORDERS

There are four major hypertensive disorders that occur in pregnant women:[5]

1. *Preeclampsia/eclampsia*: Preeclampsia (PE) refers to the syndrome of new onset of systolic blood pressure more than or equal to 140 mm Hg and/or diastolic pressure more than or equal to 90 mm Hg on 2 occasions more than 4 hours apart and proteinuria or new onset of hypertension and end-organ dysfunction with or without proteinuria, most often after

20 weeks of gestation in a previously normotensive woman. Eclampsia is diagnosed when seizures have occurred.

2. *Chronic (pre-existing) hypertension*: Chronic hypertension is defined as systolic pressure more than or equal to 140 mm Hg and/or diastolic pressure more than or equal to 90 mm Hg that antedates pregnancy or is present before the 20th week of pregnancy or persists longer than 12-week postpartum.
3. *Preeclampsia/Superimposed upon chronic hypertension*: PE—eclampsia superimposed upon chronic hypertension is diagnosed when a woman with chronic hypertension develops worsening hypertension with new onset proteinuria or other features of PE (e.g. elevated liver enzymes and low-platelet count).
4. *Gestational hypertension*: It refers to elevated blood pressure first detected after 20 weeks of gestation in the absence of proteinuria or other diagnostic features of PE.

Management of Patients with Hypertension in Diabetic Pregnancy

Glucose monitoring should be done by SMBG as optimal glycemia during pregnancy will minimize complications to the mother and the fetus. Screening, monitoring, and intervention for maternal medical comorbidities like retinopathy, nephropathy, cardiovascular system (CVS) disease, ketoacidosis, and thyroid disease should be done. Patients on angiotensin-converting enzyme (ACE) inhibitors or receptor blocker for hypertension should be taken off these medications prior to pregnancy because of their teratogenic potential. If a woman conceives while on these drugs, these should be stopped and patients may be switched over to other drugs. American Diabetes Association (ADA) suggests blood pressure targets of 120–160/85–105 mm Hg in women with chronic hypertension. In women with end-organ damage with long-standing diabetes, hypertension should be maintained less than 140/90 mm Hg to avoid progression of disease during pregnancy.

Poor glycemic control can lead to pregestational hypertension, vascular, and renal disease. Incidence of PE in diabetic women with and without vascular disease has been reported to be 17% and 8% where in women without diabetes, it is reported to be 5–8%. In a study by Holmes et al.[6] with increasing glycated hemoglobin levels, risk of preeclampsia is significantly increased.

Reason for preeclampsia with increasing HbA1C level is that insulin resistance appears to increase the risk of developing PE in the absence of overt diabetes. Impaired endothelium-dependent vasodilation depends on the duration of diabetes.

Flowchart 15.1: Hyperglycemia-induced vascular complications.

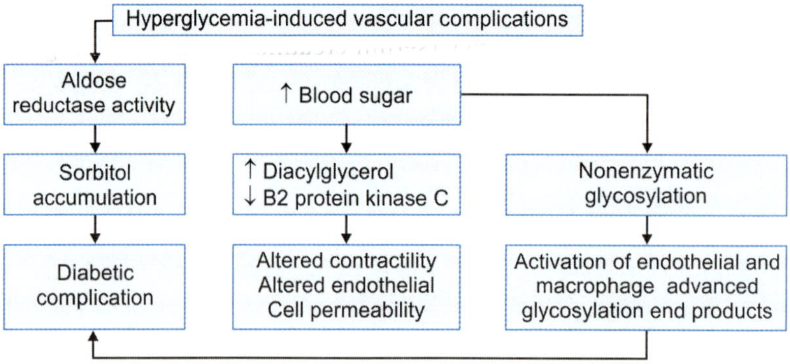

(Na–K ATP: Sodium–potassium adenosine triphosphate).

Prevention of Preeclampsia

Prenatal and first trimester: Pregestational diabetes and history of gestational diabetes in previous pregnancy is a risk factor for preeclampsia. USPST (United States Preventive Service Task) force recommends to start aspirin in beginning of second trimester and continue it till 36 weeks in these women.

Diagnosis and management of PE is similar in women with or without diabetes except in women with pre-existing nephropathy. Rates of indicated or spontaneous preterm delivery are higher in women with pregestational diabetes. Indicated preterm delivery is primarily due to PE, but other usual indications are fetal growth restriction, abruption or worsening maternal renal insufficiency or acute proliferative retinopathy.[7]

Close monitoring of women with gestational hypertension or preeclampsia without severe features is done with serial assessment of maternal symptoms and fetal movement (daily by the woman), serial measurements of BP (twice weekly), and assessment of platelet counts and liver enzymes (weekly) is suggested.[5]

Careful monitoring is required to look for features of severe PE in women with hypertension. Severe features of PE include any of the following findings:[5]

- Systolic blood pressure of 160 mm Hg or higher, or diastolic blood pressure of 110 mm Hg or higher on two occasions at least 4 hours apart while the patient is on bed rest (unless antihypertensive therapy is initiated before this time).
- Thrombocytopenia (platelet count less than 100,000/microliter).
- Impaired liver function as indicated by abnormally elevated blood concentrations of liver enzymes (to twice normal concentration).

- Severe persistent right upper quadrant or epigastric pain unresponsive to medication and not accounted for by alternative diagnoses, or both.
- Progressive renal insufficiency (serum creatinine concentration greater than 1.1 mg/dL or a doubling of the serum creatinine concentration in the absence of other renal disease)
- Pulmonary edema.
- New-onset cerebral or visual disturbances

For women with gestational hypertension or preeclampsia with a persistent BP of more than 160 mm Hg systolic or 110 mm Hg diastolic, anti-hypertensive medications should be started.

Fetal Monitoring

Ultrasound is done at 28–32 weeks of gestation to assess fetal growth and thereafter at 3–4 weeks interval. Impaired growth is more common among women with diabetic vasculopathy and/or superimposed PE. If evidence of fetal growth restriction is found in women with preeclampsia, fetoplacental assessment that includes umbilical artery Doppler velocimetry as an adjunct antenatal test is recommended.[5]

PREGESTATIONAL DIABETES AND FREQUENCY OF TESTING DURING PREGNANCY

- *HbA1C*: 4–6 weeks
- *Blood glucose*: 4–7 times daily
- *Urine ketone*: If blood glucose more than 200 mg%
- Urine protein:
  - Every visit
  - Quantitative each trimester
- *Serum creatinine*: Each trimester
- *Thyroid function test (TFT)*: Baseline
- *Eye checkup*: Baseline and as and when necessary.

Soluble fms-like tyrosine kinase 1 (sFlt/PlGF) ratio more than 85 is associated with adverse outcome and imminent delivery and perinatal outcome within 2 weeks of presentation. Abnormally high sFlt-1 levels may serve as a surrogate for glomerular endotheliosis.[8]

TIMING OF DELIVERY

For women with preeclampsia, it is suggested that the mode of delivery need not be cesarean delivery. The mode of delivery should be determined by fetal gestational age, fetal presentation, cervical status, and maternal and fetal conditions. For women with severe PE or eclampsia, the administration of parenteral magnesium sulfate is recommended.

Prior to and during pregnancy, multidisciplinary care involving obstetrician, endocrinologist, dietician, nephrologist, and cardiologist may be helpful. For women with mild gestational hypertension or preeclampsia without severe features and no indication for delivery at less than 37 0/7 weeks of gestation,[5] expectant management with maternal and fetal monitoring is suggested. For women with severe preeclampsia at or beyond 34 0/7 weeks of gestation, and in those with unstable maternal or fetal conditions irrespective of gestational age, delivery soon after maternal stabilization and corticosteroid for fetal lung maturity is recommended.[5] It is recommended that corticosteroids be given if the fetus is viable and at 33 6/7 weeks or less of gestation, but that delivery not be delayed after initial maternal stabilization regardless of gestational age for women with severe PE that is complicated further with any of the following:[5]

- Uncontrollable severe hypertension
- Eclampsia
- Pulmonary edema
- Abruptio placentae
- Disseminated intravascular coagulation
- Evidence of nonreassuring fetal status
- Intrapartum fetal demise

ANTIHYPERTENSIVE THERAPY[9] (TABLE 15.1)

Table 15.1: Antihypertensive drugs.

1. Methyldopa	α-2 adrenergic agonist and centrally acting	*Dose*: • *Oral*: 250 mg 2–3 times daily, Maximum dose 3,000 mg/day • *IV*: 250–1,000 mg 6–8 hourly, Maximum 1,000 mg every 6 hours
2. Labetalol	α- and ß-adrenergic bl[illegible] agent	• *Oral*: 100 mg twice daily, Maximum dose 2,400 mg/day • *IV*: 10–20 mg IV push over 2 minutes, maximum dose 300 mg
3. Calcium (Nifedipine) channel blockers	*CCB*: Arteriolar vasodilatation by blocking Ca channels in vascular smooth muscles	Orally 5–10 mg thrice daily

Contd...

Contd...

4. Hydralazine	Relaxes arterial smooth, muscles by peripheral vasodilatation	• *Orally*: 100 mg in four divided doses • *IV*: 5–10 mg in 20–40 minutes to a total cumulative dose of 30 mg (IM) and 20 mg IV
5. Clonidine	Centrally acting	• *Oral*: 0.1 mg twice daily (maximum recommended dose 2.4 mg/day)

(IV: Intravenous; CCB: Calcium channel blocker)

CONCLUSION

Hypertension is a common complication in diabetic pregnancies which adversely affects the maternal and perinatal outcome. It requires close monitoring and supervised management to prevent complications and achieve optimal pregnancy outcome. Blood pressure should be monitored during postpartum period and these women should be adequately counseled to prevent complications during next pregnancy and later on in life.

KEY POINTS

- Incidence of PE in diabetic women with or without vascular disease has been reported to be 17% and 8%.
- Incidence of PE increases significantly with increasing glycated hemoglobin.
- High HbA1C leading to PE is due to insulin resistance leading to impaired endothelium-dependent vasodilatation.
- Screening, monitoring, maintaining glycemic control, and intervention for maternal medical complications are the key factors in these patients.
- Angiotensin-converting enzyme inhibitors should be stopped prior to planning pregnancy, as these have teratogenic potential.
- Use of the sFlt-1/PlGF ratio for risk stratification of women undergoing PE evaluation has the potential to reduce both morbidity and healthcare cost.
- For women with mild gestational hypertension or preeclampsia without severe features and no indication for delivery at less than 37 0/7 weeks of gestation, expectant management with maternal and fetal monitoring is suggested.
- For women with severe preeclampsia at or beyond 34 0/7 weeks of gestation, and in those with unstable maternal or fetal conditions irrespective of gestational age, delivery soon after maternal stabilization and corticosteroid for fetal lung maturity is recommended.

- It is recommended that corticosteroids be given if the fetus is viable and at 33 6/7 weeks or less of gestation, but that delivery not be delayed after initial maternal stabilization regardless of gestational age for women with severe PE that is complicated further with uncontrollable severe, hypertension, eclampsia,pulmonary edema, abruptio placentae, disseminated intravascular coagulation, evidence of nonreassuring fetal status or with intrapartum fetal demise.

REFERENCES

1. Sibai BM, Caritis S, Hauth J, et al. Risks of preeclampsia and adverse neonatal outcomes among women with pregestational diabetes mellitus. National Institute of Child Health and Human Development Network of Maternal-Fetal Medicine Units. Am J Obstet Gynecol. 2000;182:364-9.
2. Innes KE, Wimsatt JH, McDuffie R. Relative glucose tolerance and subsequent development of hypertension in pregnancy. Obstet Gynecol. 2001;97:905-10.
3. Colatrella A, Braucci S, Festa C, et al. Hypertensive disorders in normal/overweight and obese type 2 diabetic pregnant women. Exp Clin Endocrinol Diabetes. 2009;117:373-7.
4. Sibai BM, Cartitis SN, Hauth JC, et al. Preterm delivery in women with pregestational diabetes mellitus or chronic hypertension relative to women with uncomplicated pregnancies. National Institute of Child Health and Human Development Network of Maternal-Fetal Medicine Units. Am J Obstet Gynecol. 2000;183:1520-4.
5. American College of Obstetricians and Gynecologists, Task Force on Hypertension in Pregnancy. Hypertension in pregnancy. Report of the American College of Obstetricians and Gynecologists' Task Force on Hypertension in Pregnancy. Obstet Gynecol. 2013;122:1122.
6. Holmes VA, Young IS, Patterson CC, et al. Optimal glycemic control, pre-eclampsia and gestational hypertension in women with type 1 diabetes in the diabetes and pre-eclampsia intervention trial. Diabetes Care. 2011;34:1683-8.
7. Acker DB, Barss VA. Obstetrical complications. In: Brown FM, Hare JW (Eds). Diabetes complication Pregnancy, 2nd edition. New York: Wiley-Liss; 1995. p 153.
8. Kleinrouweler CE, Wiegerinck MM, Ris-Stalpers C, et al. Accuracy of circulating placental growth factor, vascular endothelial growth factor, soluble fms-like tyrosine kinase 1 and soluble endoglin in the prediction of pre-eclampsia: a systematic review and meta-analysis. BJOG. 2012;119:778-87.
9. American College of Obstetricians and Gynecologists (ACOG). Hypertension in pregnancy. Report of the American College of Obstetricians and Gynecologists' Task Force on Hypertension in Pregnancy. Obstet Gynecol. 2013;122(5):1122-31.

CHAPTER 16

Antenatal Care in Diabetes in Pregnancy

Alka Pandey, Shalini Jaggi, Shalini

INTRODUCTION

Diabetes is a common medical disorder occurring in pregnancy. It has become the modern epidemic and recently India has become capital of diabetes. Increasing incidence of diabetes in pregnancy reflects increasing prevalence of obesity and metabolic syndrome due to older maternal age, adoption of modern lifestyle, changing eating habits, and reduced physical activity.

PREVALENCE

Worldwide, one in ten pregnancies is associated with diabetes, 90% of which are gestational diabetes mellitus (GDM). In India, incidence of GDM is 10–14.3%. Its incidence is expected to increase to 20%, i.e. one in every five pregnant woman is likely to have GDM.[1]

ETIOLOGICAL CLASSIFICATION OF DIABETES MELLITUS

Type 1

- Beta-cell destruction, usually absolute insulin deficiency.
- Immune mediated.
- Idiopathic.
- Young age (juvenile).

Type 2

- Ranges from predominantly insulin resistance to predominantly an insulin secretary defect with insulin resistance.
- Late age onset overweight women.

Other Types

- *Genetic mutations of beta-cell function:* Maturity onset diabetes of the young (MODY 1-6). It has autosomal dominant mode of inheritance and manifests in adulthood.
- Genetic defects in insulin action.
- *Genetic syndromes:* Down, Klinefelter, and Turner.
- *Disease of exocrine pancreas:* Pancreatitis cystic fibrosis.
- *Endocrinopathies:* Cushing syndrome, pheochromocytoma, and others.
- *Drug or chemical induced:* Glucocorticosteroids, thiazides, beta-adrenergic agonist, and others.
- *Infections:* Congenital rubella, cytomegalovirus (CMV), and coxsackie virus.

Gestational Diabetes

Any degree of impaired glucose tolerance with onset or first recognition during pregnancy.

EFFECT OF PREGNANCY ON DIABETES

- In pregnancy there is altered carbohydrate metabolism and impaired insulin action due to combined effect of human placental lactogen, estrogen, progesterone, and degradation of insulin by placenta. Hence, stabilization of glucose becomes a problem.
- Insulin requirement during pregnancy increases as pregnancy advances.
- Ketoacidosis can be precipitated during hyperemesis in early pregnancy, infection, and fasting during labor.
- Vascular changes (retinopathy, nephropathy, coronary artery disease, and neuropathy) may be worsened.
- Insulin requirement falls significantly in puerperium.

EFFECT OF DIABETES ON PREGNANCY

Adverse pregnancy outcomes occur due to diabetes.

Maternal

Abortion, preterm labor (20%), infection, preeclampsia, polyhydramnios, diabetic retinopathy, nephropathy, and ketoacidosis.

During Labor

Prolonged labor, shoulder dystocia, perineal injuries, postpartum hemorrhage (PPH), and increased operative interference.

Puerperium

Puerperal sepsis and lactation failure.

Fetal

- Macrosomia (30–40%)
- Congenital malformation (6–10%)
- Birth injuries
- Growth restriction
- Fetal death.

Neonatal

Hypoglycemia, respiratory distress syndrome, hyperbilirubinemia, polycythemia, hypocalcemia, and hypomagnesemia.

MANAGEMENT

The management of GDM must involve a team approach consisting of obstetrician, diabetes physician, a diabetes educator, dietician, midwife, and pediatrician.[2,3] The individualized treatment plan must involve a combination of glucose monitoring, medical nutrition therapy (MNT), pharmacotherapy, exercise, weight management strategies and psychological support.[2,3]

SCREENING FOR GESTATIONAL DIABETES MELLITUS (FLOWCHART 16.1)

In light of the 11-folds increased risk of developing glucose intolerance during pregnancy in Asian women compared to Caucasian women, universal screening is preferable in India.

DIAGNOSTIC CRITERIA FOR GESTATIONAL DIABETES MELLITUS (TABLE 16.1)

Diabetes in Pregnancy Study Group India (DIPSI) guideline for diagnosis of GDM, according to 75 g oral glucose tolerance test is followed in India.[4]

PRECONCEPTION COUNSELING

- It includes strict glycemic control, so as to maintain physiological level of glucose.
- Folic acid supplementation, 5 mg/day should be given until 12 weeks of gestation to reduce neural tube defect in baby.
- Therapy must be targeted to achieve prepregnancy hemoglobin A1c (HbA1c) of less than 6.5% [National Institute for Health and Care Excellence (NICE) guidelines 2008]. Those with HbA1c more than 10% should avoid pregnancy.
- Evaluation of end organ damage should be done.

Flowchart 16.1: Universal testing for gestational diabetes mellitus.

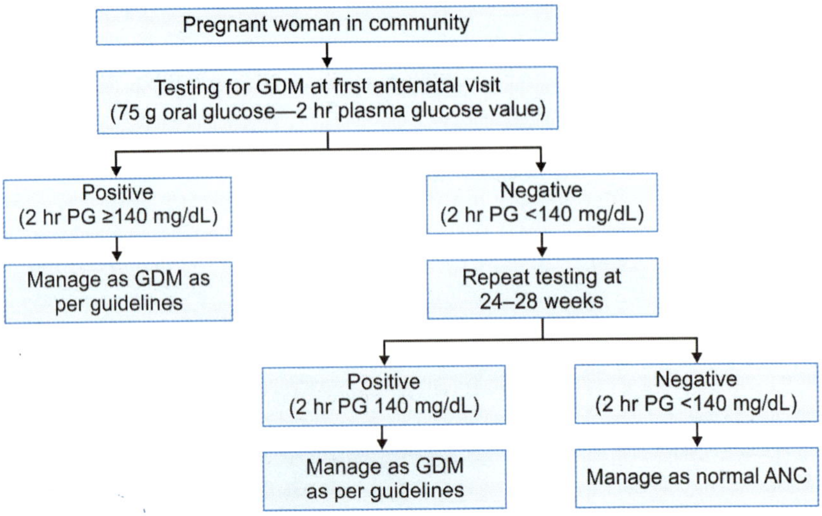

(GDM: Gestational diabetes mellitus; PG: Plasma glucose; ANC: Antenatal care)
Source: National Guidelines for Diagnosis & Management of Gestational Diabetes Mellitus.

Table 16.1: Diabetes in Pregnancy Study Group India (DIPSI) guideline for diagnosis of gestational diabetes mellitus.

Criteria	*In pregnancy*	*Outside pregnancy*
2 hr ≥ 200 mg/dL	Diabetes	Diabetes
2 hr ≥ 140 mg/dL	GDM	IGT
2 hr ≥ 120 mg/dL	DGGT	---

(GDM: Gestational diabetes mellitus; DGGT: Decreased gestational glucose tolerance; IGT: Impaired glucose tolerance).

ANTENATAL CARE

At antenatal appointments specific care is provided to women with diabetes in addition to the routine care (Flowchart 16.2).

Booking Appointments: Ideally by

10 Weeks:

- Counseling about effects of diabetes on pregnancy, diet, achieving optimum blood glucose control, birth, and early parenting.
- Measurement of HbA1c levels for women with pre-existing diabetes to determine level of risk of pregnancy.
- Viability of pregnancy should be confirmed at 7–9 weeks.

- 75 g oral glucose tolerance test should be advised to women with no pre-existing diabetes.

16 Weeks:

- Retinal assessment at 16–20 weeks in women with overt diabetes, if diabetic retinopathy was present at their first antenatal care (ANC).
- 75 g oral glucose tolerance test should be advised to women with no diabetes who book in second trimester.

20 Weeks:

- Ultrasound to detect structural abnormalities including fetal heart examination.

28 Weeks:

- Ultrasound monitoring of fetal growth and amniotic fluid volume.
- Retinal assessment of women with pre-existing diabetes.

32 Weeks:

- Ultrasound monitoring of fetal growth and amniotic fluid volume.

36 Weeks:

- Counseling about timing, management of birth, analgesia, changes in blood glucose level during and after birth, care of the baby, breastfeeding, and contraception.

37 Weeks to 38 + 6 Weeks Gestation:

- Induction of labor or caesarean should be offered, if indicated in women with type 1 or type 2 diabetes.
- *38 weeks*: Tests for fetal wellbeing [fetal umbilical artery Doppler recording, fetal heart rate (FHR) recording, and biophysical profile is

Flowchart 16.2: Management of pregnant woman with gestational diabetes mellitus.

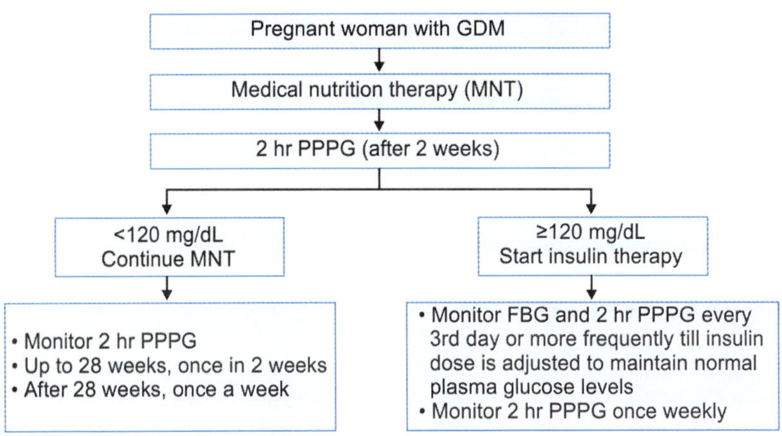

(GDM: Gestational diabetes mellitus; PPPG: Postprandial plasma glucose; FBG: Fasting blood glucose).

Source: National Guidelines for Diagnosis & Management of Gestational Diabetes Mellitus.

not recommended in pregnant women with diabetes unless there is intrauterine growth restriction (IUGR)].

- *39 weeks*: Tests for fetal wellbeing, women with uncomplicated GDM to give birth not later than 40 + 6 weeks.[5]

In pregnant women with GDM having uncontrolled blood glucose level or any other complication of pregnancy, the frequency of antenatal visits should be increased to every 2 weeks in second trimester and every week in third trimester.

Pregnant women with GDM should be monitored for hypertension in pregnancy, proteinuria, and other obstetric complications.

In pregnant women with GDM between 24 weeks and 34 weeks of gestation and requiring early delivery, antenatal steroids should be given. Dexamethasone 6 mg intramuscular (IM) 12 hourly for 2 days. More vigilant monitoring of blood glucose levels should be done for next 72 hours and the dose of insulin should be adjusted accordingly.[1]

Fetal Surveillance

- Fundal height, abdominal girth, maternal weight gain daily fetal movement count and fetal heart sound should be monitored at each visit to evaluate fetal growth.
- Serial USG, NST, biophysical profile and doppler study may be done as required.
- *Daily fetal activity assessment*: The women should lie down on her side after a meal and note how long it takes for the fetus to kick 10 times. If the fetus does not kick 10 times within 2 hours, she should immediately consult her health care provider.

Medical Nutrition Therapy—First Line Therapy

- Done in consultation with nutritionist in account with dietary habits and cultural preferences.
- Calories intake should consist of less than 45% carbohydrates, 30% protein, and 25% fat (unsaturated).
- Carbohydrate should be spread in three small meals and 2–3 snacks.
- Complex carbohydrate should be preferred over simple ones.
- High fiber diet may help in controlling blood sugar by delaying gastric emptying.
- A woman of body mass index (BMI) less than 25 kg/m^2—needs 3,000 calories/day, overweight (BMI 25–30 kg/m^2)—needs 2,500 calories/day, and morbidly obese (BMI >40 kg/m^2)—needs 1,250 calories/day.
- Calorie must be met through three major and three minor meals at equal intervals.

Exercise

- 30 minutes of mild to moderate exercise daily helps to improve glycemic control by improving insulin sensitivity at skeletal muscle level.
- Walking after meal reduces postprandial (PP) glucose levels.
- There is insufficient evidence to recommend or advice against pregnant women with GDM enrolling in exercise programs.
- Even if exercise is not beneficial during pregnancy this change in life style may be continued after delivery and may help to prevent the onset of type 2 diabetes and its long-term complications.

Pharmacotherapy

Insulin Therapy (Flowchart 16.3)

It has been considered gold standard in treatment of diabetes in pregnancy. Rapid acting insulin analogues (aspart and lispro) have advantage over long acting ones. Injection human premix insulin 30/70 is recommended by National guidelines.

Refer to higher center, if one or more of the following conditions are met:

- Excessive nausea and vomiting.
- Fasting blood glucose >200 mg/dL with or without insulin.
- Fasting blood glucose >150 mg/dL or post breakfast >250 mg/dL even after giving insulin.
- Total dose of insulin (combined morning and evening dose) on each day exceeds 20 units.
- If pregnant women develops low blood glucose (hypoglycemia) more than once in a day.
- If pregnant woman refuses to take insulin injection.

How to Recognize and Manage Hypoglycemia

- Any pregnant woman on insulin can develop hypoglycemia at any time.
- Hypoglycemia is diagnosed when blood glucose level is <70 mg/dL.
- It is important to teach the woman to recognize symptoms of hypoglycemia and treat immediately.

How to Recognize Hypoglycemia?

- *Early symptoms:* Tremors of hands, sweating, palpitations, hunger, easy fatigability, headache, mood changes, irritability, low attentiveness, tingling sensation around the mouth/lips, or any other abnormal feeling.
- *Severe:* Confusion, abnormal behavior or both, visual disturbances, nervousness or anxiety, and abnormal behavior.
- *Uncommon:* Seizures and loss of consciousness.

Flowchart 16.3: Insulin therapy for pregnant woman with gestational diabetes mellitus.

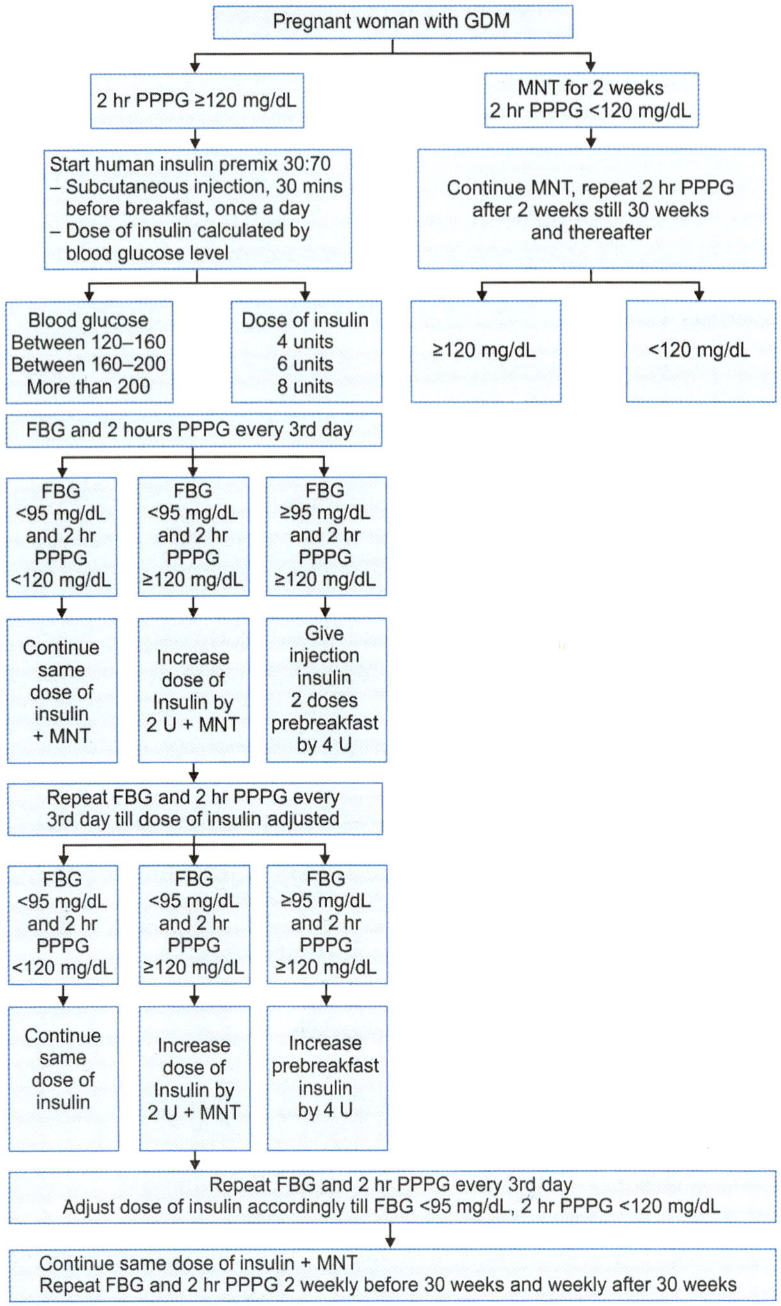

*Only injection human premix insulin 30/70 to be used, *Insulin syringe—40 IU syringe, *Subcutaneous injection only

(GDM: Gestational diabetes mellitus; PPPG: Postprandial plasma glucose; FBG: Fasting blood glucose; MNT: Medical nutrition therapy).

Source: National Guidelines for Diagnosis & Management of Gestational Diabetes Mellitus.

How to Manage Hypoglycemia?

- Ask pregnant woman to take 3 TSF of glucose powder (15–20 g) dissolved in a glass of water.
- After taking oral glucose, she must take rest and avoid any physical activity.
- 15 minutes after taking glucose, she must eat one chapati with vegetable/ rice/one glass of milk/idli/fruits/anything eatable which is available.
- If hypoglycemia continues, repeat same amount of glucose and wait.
- If glucose is not available, take one of the following: Sugar—6 TSF in a glass of water/fruit juice/honey/anything which is sweet/any food.
- Take rest, eat regularly, and check blood glucose, if possible.
- If PW develops >1 episode of hypoglycemia in a day, she should consult any doctor immediately.

Blood Glucose Targets and Monitoring

Recommendation for blood glucose monitoring:
- Fasting plasma glucose (FPG) and 2 hours PP peak levels around 90 mg/dL and 120 mg/dL, respectively are recommended as blood glucose targets in patients with GDM.
- Titration of dose should be based on self-monitoring of blood glucose (SMBG): 7 tests/day, 3 before and 3 after each meal and 1 at 3 am. As a compromise 1 fasting and 3 each after breakfast, lunch and dinner at least twice a week is more feasible and acceptable.[4]

INSULIN PEN

Recommendations for Insulin Therapy Using Insulin Pens

Insulin pens are recommended to make the injections accurate, discreet, and painless with successful self-administration (grade A; EL 2).[4]

Recommendations for Insulin Therapy Using Insulin Pumps

Continuous subcutaneous insulin therapy is recommended in patients with GDM and pre-GDM for achieving euglycemia when warranted. However, it is not recommended as a part of routine practice (grade A; EL 2).[4]

ORAL ANTIDIABETIC DRUGS

Recent studies have indicated that there may be beneficial effects associated with the use of metformin and glyburide during pregnancy.[6,7] On the other hand significant concerns remain about the use of oral antidiabetic agents (OADs) during pregnancy, primarily due to safety issues.[8,9] Oral antidiabetic agents have been discussed in details in another chapter.

KEY POINTS

- Universal testing of all PW for diabetes should be done.
- Testing is recommended twice in pregnancy at first antenatal visit and then at 24–28 weeks of gestation and then after 30 weeks.
- Single step 75 g 2-hr postprandial plasma glucose (PPPG) test is performed.
- Pregnant women testing positive (2-hr PPPG >140 mg/dL) should be started on MNT for 2 weeks.
- If 2-hr PPPG ≥120 mg/dL after MNT, medical management (insulin therapy) of pregnant women should be started as per guidelines.
- Pregnant women should be monitored by 2-hr PPPG throughout pregnancy as per guidelines.
- Antenatal visits 2 weekly in second trimester and weekly in third trimester.
- Pregnant women with GDM on insulin therapy with uncontrolled blood glucose levels (2-hr PPPG ≥120 mg/dL) or insulin requirement >20 U/day should be referred for delivery at higher centers.
- GDM pregnancies are associated with delay in lung maturity of the fetus; so routine delivery prior to 39 weeks is not recommended.
- Early delivery with administration of prophylactic corticosteroid therapy for fetal lung maturity is to be planned only if uncontrolled plasma glucose or any other obstetric indication is there.
- Vaginal delivery is preferred; lower segment cesarean section (LSCS) should be done for only obstetric indications or fetal macrosomia.
- Neonatal monitoring for hypoglycemia and other complications should be done carefully.
- Postpartum evaluation of glycemic status by a 75 g oral glucose tolerance test (OGTT) at 6 weeks after delivery should be done.

REFERENCES

1. Maternal Health Division, Ministry of Health and Family Welfare, Government of India. (2014). National Guidelines for Diagnosis & Management of Gestational Diabetes Mellitus. [online] Available from http://www.nrhmorissa.gov.in/writereaddata/Upload/Documents/National%20Guidelines%20for%20Diagnosis%20&%20Management%20of%20Gestational%20Diabetes%20Mellitus.pdf [Accessed December 2017].
2. Castorino K, Jovanovič L. Pregnancy and diabetes management: advances and controversies. Clin Chem. 2011;57(2):221-30.
3. Mathiesen ER, Ringholm L, Damm P. Pregnancy management of women with pregestational diabetes. Endocrinol Metab Clin North Am. 2011;40:727-38.
4. Seshiah V, Banerjee S, Balaji V, et al. Consensus evidence-based guidelines for management of gestational diabetes mellitus in India. J Assoc Physicians India. 2014;62(7 Suppl):55-62.

5. NICE. (2015). Diabetes in pregnancy: management from preconception to the postnatal period. [online] Available from https://www.nice.org.uk/guidance/ng3 [Accessed December 2017].
6. Gui J, Liu Q, Feng L. Metformin vs insulin in the management of gestational diabetes: a meta-analysis. PLoS One. 2013;8(5):e64585.
7. Joy S, Roman A, Istwan N, et al. The effect of maternal obesity on pregnancy outcomes of women with gestational diabetes controlled with diet only, glyburide, or insulin. Am J Perinatol. 2012;29:643-8.
8. Hellmuth E, Damm P, Mølsted-Pedersen L. Oral hypoglycaemic agents in 118 diabetic pregnancies. Diabet Med. 2000;17:507-11.
9. Cheng YW, Chung JH, Block-Kurbisch I, et al. Treatment of gestational diabetes mellitus: glyburide compared to subcutaneous insulin therapy and associated perinatal outcomes. J Matern Fetal Neonatal Med. 2012;25:379-84.

CHAPTER 17

Challenges in the Management of Macrosomia in Diabetic Pregnancy

Pikee Saxena, Abha Singh, Raksha Soni

INTRODUCTION

The American College of Obstetricians and Gynecologists (ACOG) defined macrosomia as birth-weight over 4,500 g irrespective of gestational age or greater than the 90th percentile for gestational age after correcting for neonatal sex and ethnicity.[1] Macrosomia affects 3–15% of all pregnancies.[2]

RISK FACTORS

According to the ACOG committee, the risk factors for fetal macrosomia other than pre-existing diabetes mellitus in decreasing order of importance are—previous history of macrosomia, prepregnancy maternal weight, weight gain during pregnancy, multiparity, male fetus, gestational age more than 40 weeks, ethnicity, maternal birth weight, maternal height, and a positive 50 g glucose screen with a negative result on the 3-hour glucose tolerance test. These risk factors including genetics have been studied in various studies in relation to macrosomia.[3-5] It has been observed that fetuses of obese women with gestational diabetes mellitus have a higher risk of developing macrosomia than those of nonobese women with gestational diabetes mellitus.

PATHOPHYSIOLOGY

Intermittent periods of hyperglycemia are common with poorly controlled diabetes, maternal obesity, and excessive maternal weight gain. Maternal hyperglycemia leads to hyperglycemia in the fetus causing stimulation of fetal pancreas to secrete insulin, insulin-like growth factors, growth hormone, and other growth factors, which stimulate fetal growth and deposition of fat and glycogen. Advancing gestational age causes continued in utero growth resulting in larger birth weight at delivery.

Data from the Diabetes in Early Pregnancy Study indicate that fetal birth weight correlates best with second- and third-trimester postprandial blood sugar levels and not with fasting or mean-glucose levels.[6] When postprandial glucose values average 120 mg/dL or less, approximately 20% of infants can be expected to be macrosomic, and if the glucose values are as high as 160 mg/dL, the rate of macrosomia can reach up to 35%.

On the other hand, data from the Australian Carbohydrate Intolerance Study (ACHOIS) in Pregnant Women demonstrated a positive relationship between the severity of maternal fasting hyperglycemia and the risk of shoulder dystocia, with a 1 mmol increase in fasting glucose leading to a 2.09 relative risk for shoulder dystocia.[7]

Macrosomic fetuses in diabetic pregnancies develop a unique pattern of overgrowth, involving the central deposition of subcutaneous fat in the abdominal and interscapular areas.[8] They have larger shoulder and extremity circumferences, a decreased head-to-shoulder ratio, significantly higher body fat, and thicker upper-extremity skinfolds.

DIAGNOSIS

There is no standardized algorithm for performing antenatal monitoring of fetal macrosomia. Concept of use of percentile makes the diagnosis of macrosomia independent of gestational age, but confusion is created when different authors use 90th, 95th, or 97th percentile or 2 SD above median to define macrosomia. Gender-specific values should be considered, as males are heavier than females.

Weighing the newborn after delivery is the only way to accurately diagnose macrosomia, as the prenatal diagnostic methods including assessment of maternal risk factors, clinical examination and ultrasonographic measurement of the fetus remain imprecise.

Prediction by Clinical Examination

As per ACOG, Leopold's maneuvers and measurement of the symphysis-fundal height are the two primary methods for the clinical estimation of fetal weight. Fundal height measurement alone or in combination with symphysis-fundal height measurement has a sensitivity of 10–43% and a positive predictive value of 28–53% for fetal macrosomia diagnosis.[9,10] Poor sensitivity of clinical methods may be due to abnormal fetal lie, variation in amount of liquor, maternal obesity, lack of experienced obstetricians, or an inconsistently defined fixed point of the fundus.

Prediction by Ultrasonography

Use of prenatal ultrasound (USG) has largely replaced clinical diagnosis for macrosomia.

Ultrasound measurement of fetal abdominal circumference (AC) detects high- and low-fetal weights better than clinical examination.[11] However, it remains problematic, as the fetus has an irregular three-dimensional body of varying density and tissue composition. Hansmann[12] stated that the umbilical vein should be visualized at the level of the portal sinus otherwise the AC will be overestimated. The AC is measured at the outer surface of the skin line.[13]

A sonographic AC of more than or equal to 35 cm at the due date has a 93% positive predictive value for birth weight more than 4,000 g.[14] Repeated measurement of fetal AC led to prediction of a birth weight above the 90th percentile with 84% sensitivity and 100% specificity.[15,16] Fetal USG provides biometric data that is used to estimate the fetal weight. As compared to others, the Hadlock formula I has the smallest mean absolute error of 8.6%.[17] Sensitivity of sonographic diagnosis of fetal macrosomia (birth weight >4,000 g) varies from 12% to 75% and the specificity from 68% to 99% when different formulae for weight estimation are used.[18] The real birth weight is often underestimated when using biometric formulae to determine the estimated fetal weight.[19,20]

Recently Lee et al. observed that precision of fetal weight estimation can be improved by adding 3-dimensional USG fractional limb volume measurements to conventional 2-dimensional biometry. They demonstrated that new models, which utilize fractional limb volume may offer novel insight into the contribution of soft tissue development to fetal weight estimation.[21] Subcutaneous fat deposition at the upper arm, shoulder, thigh, and abdomen also plays a role in the body composition of the fetus and should be measured for better prediction of fetal weight.

First trimester USG screening for predicting macrosomia is also being evaluated. Plasencia et al. observed that the best predictive models for fetal birth weight included uterine artery-pulsatility index (PI), pregnancy-associated plasma protein A (PAPPA), nuchal translucency (NT), parity, maternal age, smoking status, weight, height, and free β-hCG. Pregnancies delivering newborns with macrosomia were compared with nonmacrosomic pregnancies and it was found that PAPPA and NT thickness were found to be significantly increased ($P = 0.016$ and 0.001, respectively) and uterine artery-PI was significantly decreased ($P = 0.011$). In their study, it was seen that a combination of maternal factors with PAPPA, fetal NT, and uterine artery-PI identified 34.4% of large for gestational age (LGA) newborns for a false-positive rate of 10%.[22]

Size of placenta in early pregnancy has also been found to be associated with fetal macrosomia.[23]

Drawbacks of Sonographic Methods

Three-dimensional USG is time-consuming and not widely available. Body composition is ignored by all formulae for fetal weight estimation. Other limiting factors are suboptimal views with oligohydramnios, maternal obesity, multiple pregnancies, or unfavorable fetal lie; a lack of experienced examiners; intra- and interobserver variability, outdated USG machines, and fetal anomalies, such as gastroschisis, omphalocoele, and hydrocephalus that lead to changes in biometric measurements.

It is recommended that serial USG with at least a gap of 2 weeks should occur between USG measurements and, if possible, the same sonographer should perform the examination.

COMPLICATIONS

Fetal macrosomia is associated with a number of maternal and perinatal complications. Maternal complications include infection, postpartum hemorrhage, prolonged labor, high-degree perineal tears, cesarean delivery, anesthetic accidents, and thromboembolic events.[24]

According to the American College of Obstetricians and Gynecology (ACOG), practice bulletin macrosomic fetuses have a greater risk for perinatal asphyxia, meconium aspiration, clavicular fracture, brachial plexus injury, and shoulder dystocia.[1] Shoulder dystocia represents the most serious complication associated with fetal macrosomia. Odds ratio of shoulder dystocia is 21 for fetal weight more than or equal to 4,500 g as compared for normal weight individuals. Infants with macrosomia are at increased risk of developing hypertension, obesity, and transgenerational risk of type 2 diabetes mellitus in adulthood.[25]

The perinatal mortality rate in newborns with birth weights more than 4,500 g is double than that of normal-weight babies.[26] Birth weight more than 4,000 g carries double the risk of postpartum hemorrhage of more than 1,000 mL.[27] Pregnant patients with known fetal macrosomia (4,000–4,500 g) have 4.5-fold increased risk of fourth-degree perineal tears.[28]

CLINICAL MANAGEMENT OF THE FETUS WITH MACROSOMIA

In suspected fetal macrosomia, the best mode of delivery is still being debated. In principle, the three choices of induction of labor, expectant management or elective cesarean delivery are well known.

There are conflicting results about the advantage of labor induction. A Cochrane analysis and a systematic review stated that labor induction for suspected fetal macrosomia results in an increased cesarean delivery rate without improving perinatal outcomes.[29,30] This is because the fetal lung maturity may be delayed till about 38 + 6 weeks in diabetic pregnancy as compared to normal pregnancies where lung maturity occurs by 34–35 weeks. The other reason is poor bishops in preterm induction of labor. On the other hand, in a retrospective study Cheng et al.[31] found that induction of labor may reduce the risk of cesarean delivery compared with expectant management. The patient's obstetric history, her progress during labor, and other evidence of fetopelvic disproportion should be taken into account when individually counseling about the mode of delivery in suspected fetal macrosomia.

CONCLUSION

Clinical assessment and ultrasound prediction of macrosomia are both imprecise. Macrosomia creates problems during delivery and also predisposes the fetus to metabolic diseases later in life due to intrauterine programming. Therefore, the best way to manage fetal overgrowth is to prevent it by achieving optimal glycemia.[32,33]

KEY POINTS BASED ON ACOG RECOMMENDATIONS:[1]

- The diagnosis of fetal macrosomia is imprecise. For suspected fetal macrosomia, the accuracy of estimated fetal weight using USG biometry is no better than that obtained with clinical palpation (Leopold's maneuvers). *(Level A)*
- Suspected fetal macrosomia is not an indication for induction of labor, because induction does not improve maternal or fetal outcomes. *(Level B)*
- Labor and vaginal deliveries are not contraindicated for women with estimated fetal weights up to 5,000 g in the absence of maternal diabetes. *(Level B)*
- With an estimated fetal weight more than 4,500 g, a prolonged second stage of labor or arrest of descent in the second stage is an indication for cesarean delivery. *(Level B)*
- Although the diagnosis of fetal macrosomia is imprecise, prophylactic cesarean delivery may be considered for suspected fetal macrosomia with estimated fetal weights of more than 5,000 g in pregnant women without diabetes and more than 4,500 g in pregnant women with diabetes. *(Level C)*
- Suspected fetal macrosomia is not a contraindication to attempted vaginal birth after a previous cesarean delivery. *(Level C)*
- Neonates of a diabetic mother should undergo a full physical examination from head to toe, congenital anomalies (congenital heart defects, tracheo-esophageal fistula, and central nervous system abnormalities), and birth trauma should be critically evaluated. These newborns should receive intensive observation and care and should be examined for hypoglycemia, polycythemia, hyperbilirubinemia, and electrolyte abnormalities.[34]
- The blood glucose level should be examined within 1 hour of birth and then repeated as needed. Oral feeding, ideally breastfeeding, is recommended as soon as possible, and if oral feeding is insufficient, an intravenous infusion of glucose should be started.[34]

REFERENCES

1. American College of Obstetricians and Gynecologists. Fetal macrosomia AC Washington (DC): The College of Obstetricians and Gynecologists. Practice Bulletin No 22. 2000.
2. Ventura SJ, Martin JA, Curtin SC, et al. Births: final data for 1998. Natl Vital Stat Rep. 2000;48:1-100.
3. Asplund CA, Seehusen DA, Callahan TL, et al. Percentage change in antenatal body mass index as a predictor of neonatal macrosomia. Ann Fam Med. 2008;6:550-4.
4. Abolfazl M, Hamidreza TS, Narges MY. Gestational diabetes and its association with unpleasant outcomes of pregnancy. Pak J Med Sci. 2008;24:566-70.
5. Ludwig DS, Currie J. The association between pregnancy weight gain and birth weight: a within family comparison. Lancet. 2010;376:984-90.
6. Jovanovic-Peterson L, Peterson CM, Reed GF, et al. Maternal postprandial glucose levels and infant birth weight: the Diabetes in Early Pregnancy Study. The National Institute of Child Health and Human Development—Diabetes in Early Pregnancy Study. Am J Obstet Gynecol. 1991;164:103-11.
7. Athukorala C, Crowther CA, Willson K. Women with gestational diabetes mellitus in the ACHOIS trial: risk factors for shoulder dystocia. Aust N Z J Obstet Gynaecol. 2007;47:37-41.
8. McFarland MB, Trylovich CG, Langer O. Anthropometric differences in macrosomic infants of diabetic and nondiabetic mothers. J Matern Fetal Med. 1998;7:292-5.
9. American College of Obstetricians and Gynecologists. ACOG Practice Bulletin Fetal Macrosomia. 2000.
10. O'Reilly-Green C, Divon M. Sonographic and clinical methods in the diagnosis of macrosomia. Clin Obstet Gynecol. 2000;43:309-20.
11. Kayem G, Grange G, Breart G, et al. Comparison of fundal height measurement and sonographically measured fetal abdominal circumference in the prediction of high and low birth weight at term. Ultrasound Obstet Gynecol. 2009;34:566-71.
12. Hansmann M. Ultraschallbiometrieim II. und III. Trimester der Schwangerschaft. Gynäkologe. 1976;9:133-55.
13. Salomon LJ, Alfirevic Z, Berghella V, et al. Practice guidelines for performance of the routine mid-trimester fetal ultrasound scan. Ultrasound Obstet Gynecol. 2011;37: 116-26.
14. Jazayeri A, Heffron JA, Phillips R, et al. Macrosomia prediction using ultrasound fetal abdominal circumference of 35 centimeters or more. Obstet Gynecol. 1999;93:523-6.
15. Hedriana HL, Moore TR. A comparison of single versus multiple growth ultrasonographic examinations in predicting birth weight. Am J Obstet Gynecol. 1994;170: 1600-4.
16. Coomarasamy A, Connock M, Thornton J, et al. Accuracy of ultrasound biometry in the prediction of macrosomia: a systematic quantitative review. BJOG. 2005;112: 1461-6.
17. Pinette MG, Pan Y, Pinette SG, et al. Estimation of fetal weight: mean value from multiple formulas. J Ultrasound Med. 1999;18:813-7.
18. Chauhan SP, Grobman WA, Gherman RA, et al. Suspicion and treatment of the macrosomic fetus: a review. Am J Obstet Gynecol. 2005;193:332-46.
19. Dudley NJ. A systematic review of the ultrasound estimation of fetal weight. Ultrasound Obstet Gynecol. 2005;25:80-9.
20. Scioscia M, Vimercati A, Ceci O, et al. Estimation of birth weight by two-dimensional ultrasonography: a critical appraisal of its accuracy. Obstet Gynecol 2008;111:57-65.

21. Lee W, Balasubramaniam M, Deter RL, et al. New fetal weight estimation models using fractional limb volume. Ultrasound Obstet Gynecol. 2009;34:556-65.
22. Plasencia W, González Dávila E, Tetilla V, et al. First-trimester screening for large-for-gestational-age infants. Ultrasound Obstet Gynecol. 2012;39:389-95.
23. Schwartz AN, Quant HS, Sammel MD, et al. Macrosomia has its roots in early placental development. Placenta. 2014;35(9):684-90.
24. Boulet SL, Alexander GR, Salihu HM, et al. Macrosomic births in the United States: determinants, outcomes, and proposed grades of risk. Am J Obstet Gynecol. 2003;188(5):1372-8.
25. Hermann GM, Dallas LM, Haskell SE, et al. Neonatal macrosomia is an independent risk factor for adult metabolic syndrome. Neonatology. 2010;98:238-44.
26. Modanlou HD, Dorchester WL, Thorosian A, et al. Macrosomia—maternal, fetal, and neonatal implications. Obstet Gynecol. 1980;55:420-4.
27. Stones RW, Paterson CM, Saunders NJ. Risk factors for major obstetric haemorrhage. Eur J Obstet Gynecol Reprod Biol. 1993;48:15-8.
28. Stotland NE, Caughey AB, Breed EM, et al. Risk factors and obstetric complications associated with macrosomia. Int J Gynaecol Obstet. 2004;87:220-6.
29. Irion O, Boulvain M. Induction of labour for suspected fetal macrosomia. Cochrane Database Syst Rev. 2000;CD000938.
30. Sanchez-Ramos L, Bernstein S, Kaunitz AM. Expectant management versus labor induction for suspected fetalmacrosomia: a systematic review. Obstet Gynecol. 2002;100:997-1002.
31. Cheng YW, Sparks TN, Laros RK Jr, et al. Impending macrosomia: will induction of labour modify the risk of caesarean delivery? BJOG. 2012;119:402-9.
32. Althuizen E, van Poppel MN, Seidell JC, et al. Design of the New Life(style) study: a randomised controlled trial to optimise maternal weight development during pregnancy. BMC Public Health. 2006;6:168.
33. Sandmire HF, Woolley RJ. Macrosomia: can we prevent big problems with big babies? Birth. 1998;25:263-7.
34. Athukorala C, Crowther CA, Willson K. Women with gestational diabetes mellitus in the ACHOIS trial: risk factors for shoulder dystocia. Aust N Z J Obstet Gynaecol. 2007;47:37-41.

CHAPTER 18

Fetal Monitoring in Pregnancy with Diabetes

Archana Mishra, Pikee Saxena

INTRODUCTION

Diabetes mellitus is known to complicate 6–9% of all pregnancies worldwide.[1] In India, prevalence of gestational diabetes mellitus (GDM) varies from region to region. It is reported 3.8% in Kashmir to as high as 41% in Uttar Pradesh.[2,3] At any point of time an estimated 4 million pregnancies are complicated with diabetes in India.[4] Pregnancies complicated with diabetes are at high risk for first trimester pregnancy loss, congenital anomalies, aneuploidy, macrosomia, intrauterine growth restriction (IUGR), preterm delivery (both spontaneous and iatrogenic), premature rupture of membranes, and stillbirth. Neonates suffer birth trauma, hypoglycemia, hypocalcemia, hyperbilirubinemia, polycythemia, and consequences of prematurity and congenital malformations.[5] Congenital anomalies contribute to 50% of prenatal mortality and half of it are due to cardiac abnormalities.[6] In second and third trimester, uncontrolled blood sugars may lead to macrosomia in fetus. Hyperinsulinemia in fetus due to beta cell hypertrophy may cause hypokalemia and cardiac arrhythmia. Worst outcome is intrauterine or perinatal demise. Even in later life these offsprings are prone to obesity, diabetes mellitus, and metabolic syndrome. Maintaining maternal plasma glucose levels within the euglycemic range in pregestational period and throughout the pregnancy and monitoring of fetus are the two essential elements of management of a diabetic pregnancy. Adverse perinatal outcome is reported to be decreased from 4% to 1% with adequate glycemic control.[7]

FIRST TRIMESTER SCAN

In women with pregestational diabetes, risk of early pregnancy loss is as high as 29% which can be brought down to 9% by maintaining euglycemic status.[8] Earliest first trimester scan is desirable for viability and correct dating of pregnancy especially in cases where menstrual history is not reliable. A subset of these patients is suffering from polycystic ovarian syndrome or hypothyroidism and has irregular menstrual cycle. Accurate dating is essential while timing the termination of pregnancy. Other advantages of early scan are detection of undiagnosed missed abortion and multiple pregnancy. Scans performed in second and third trimester are less accurate due to chances of macrosomia. Early growth delay detected in first trimester scan done at 9–11 weeks is associated with a seven times increased incidence of congenital anomaly in fetus.[9] Uncontrolled blood sugar in early pregnancy, especially in first trimester during the period of organogenesis, is particularly detrimental for the fetus as it is teratogenic for the developing cells. Risk of congenital malformation is increased by threefold as compared to general population. Hypoglycemia in early pregnancy has been excluded as a cause of embryopathy, but other probable reasons for embryopathy are genetic predisposition, ketonemia, fetal zinc depletion, and inhibited somatomedin action.[10] Ultrasound at this gestation can detect central nervous system (CNS) abnormalities, such as anencephaly with fair accuracy.

EARLY ANEUPLOIDY SCREENING

All the women of pregestational diabetes should be offered aneuploidy screening. First trimester aneuploidy screening done from 11 weeks to 13 + 6 weeks includes measurement of maternal serum pregnancy-associated plasma protein A (PAPP-A), beta human chorionic gonadotropin (hCG) (either free or total) in collaboration with nuchal translucency on ultrasound done at crown rump length of approximately 38–84 mm. Results are combined with maternal age to compute aneuploidy risk and perceived risk of anomaly. Patient should also be educated on the options of screening and diagnostic testing in pregnancy, such as cell free deoxyribonucleic acid (DNA) testing, chorionic villus sampling, or amniocentesis. Most recent studies reported a decreased median levels of PAPP-A and free beta hCG in pregestational diabetes and need for correction factor in screening.[11]

SECOND TRIMESTER ANEUPLOIDY SCREENING

Second trimester risk assessment includes quadruple test that analyze unconjugated estriol (uE3), beta hCG, and dimeric inhibin A along with maternal serum alpha-fetoprotein. This along with anomaly scan at 18–20 weeks has highest detection rate of 90% with only 2% false positive rate. Maternal factors such as diabetes mellitus, weight, race, parity, multiple gestation, smoking, and in vitro fertilization are reported to affect the detection rate and false positive rate of screening for aneuploidy. Maternal serum alpha-fetoprotein is decreased in pregnancies affected by diabetes. A correction factor of 10–20% upward adjustment is used by most laboratories.[12]

SECOND TRIMESTER ANOMALY SCAN

Second trimester detailed anomaly scan has to be performed at 18–20 weeks of gestation to rule out anomalies of CNS, cardiovascular system (CVS), skeletal system, genitourinary system, etc. Soft markers for aneuploidy are to be assessed simultaneously. Following anomalies are encountered in pregnancies with diabetes. Cardiac anomalies which are common include transposition of the great vessels, ventricular septal defects, atrial septal defects, coarctation of the aorta, cardiomyopathy, and single umbilical artery. Common anomalies of CNS are anencephaly, spina bifida, microcephaly, and holoprosencephaly. Damage of skeletal system causes caudal regression syndrome, sacral agenesis, and limb defects. Renal anomalies are renal agenesis, hydronephrosis, and ureteric abnormalities. Common gastrointestinal system anomalies are duodenal atresia, anorectal atresia, and small left colon syndrome.

FETAL ECHOCARDIOGRAPHY

Although in majority of cases, a morphologically normal looking four chamber view of fetal heart with visualization of great vessels is enough. Fetal echo can be offered at 18–24 weeks in high-risk cases, such as:

- Suspected cardiac anomaly on scan
- Presence of other anomalies
- Positive aneuploidy screening
- Compromised visibility due to maternal obesity
- Pregestational diabetes with uncontrolled blood sugars
- History of drug intake like antiepileptics
- Rubella in index pregnancy or
- History of congenital heart disease in family.

FETAL TESTING

Third trimester is considered critical for pregnancies complicated with diabetes. Women on insulin therapy especially with uncontrolled blood sugars are at high risk of stillbirth. Probable causes of sudden intrauterine death in diabetic pregnancy are fetal anaerobic metabolism leading to fetal hypoxia, acidosis, hypokalemia leading to dysrhythmias, placental insufficiency, and fluctuant supply of essential nutrients.[13] Strong association is observed between fasting hyperglycemia (> 105 mg/dL or 5.8 mmol/L) with increase in the risk of intrauterine fetal death after 32 weeks of pregnancy.[14] Chances of adverse maternal and fetal outcome can be reduced by strict glucose control and antenatal fetal testing.[7] There are lack of consensus and prevalence of wide range of practices regarding the timing and modalities of fetal surveillance.[15] Fetal surveillance depends on glycemic status and presence of other risk factors for adverse pregnancy outcomes, e.g. advanced maternal age, previous stillbirth and comorbidities, such as chronic hypertension, nephropathy, or preeclampsia. Considering severity of disease patients can broadly be classified into:

- Diet controlled GDM
- Pregestational diabetes or GDM on pharmacotherapy [insulin/oral hypoglycemic agent (OHA)].

American College of Obstetricians and Gynecologists Guidelines (2013 and 2017)[16,17]

Diet-controlled Gestational Diabetes Mellitus

These are the patients in which blood sugar levels are well within range with diet and exercise alone and there is no other pregnancy complication such as macrosomia, preeclampsia, IUGR, polyhydramnios, or oligohydramnios. Risk of stillbirth in this subset is equal to the general population, so it is reasonable to follow fetal monitoring according to local practice patterns for other low-risk pregnancies. If fetal growth and liquor volume are appropriate for gestational age on clinical examination, these pregnancies can be monitored by daily fetal movement count starting from 30 weeks to 32 weeks. Any decrease in fetal movements should be reported immediately and managed by further testing. Fetal monitoring can be initiated closer or at term.

Pregestational Diabetes or Gestational Diabetes Mellitus on Pharmacotherapy (Insulin/Oral Hypoglycemic Agent)

These are those patients who require insulin or oral hypoglycemic agents to maintain euglycemic level or who have poorly controlled blood sugar levels. Such pregnancies should be monitored intensively. Baseline fetal biometry should be done at 28 weeks along with risk assessment for macrosomia in later gestation. Biometry should be repeated at every 3–4 weeks till termination of pregnancy. Fetal growth and liquor volume is a reflection of blood sugar control of patient. Fetal testing should be done by nonstress test (NST), amniotic fluid index (AFI), or biophysical profile (BPP) alone or in combination weekly from 32 weeks to 36 weeks. 36 weeks onwards frequency can be increased to twice weekly considering high risk of stillbirth. In presence of complicating factors, such as macrosomia, polyhydramnios, IUGR, oligohydramnios, preeclampsia, etc. fetal testing should be started at an early gestation around 28 weeks.[17] Frequency of monitoring may be increased according to dynamic status of patient.

The Canadian Task Force on Preventative Health Care (2016) has also summarized an evidence-based approach of antenatal fetal testing in pregnancy with diabetes. Salient points of this guideline are:

- Fetal biometry should be started at 28 weeks as a base line and repeated every 3–4 weekly to assess the correlation between maternal glycemic control and fetal growth including amniotic fluid volume *(Evidence level II-2B).*

- 36 weeks onwards for pregestational diabetes mellitus, gestational diabetes and for even the diet controlled GDM, weekly NST, AFI, and BPP either alone or in combination is recommended *(Evidence level III A)*.
- Fetal surveillance may be started early and may be done twice weekly in setting of complicating factors like obesity, uncontrolled blood sugars, proven macrosomia, previous history of stillbirth, preeclampsia, or IUGR *(Evidence level II-2A)*.

Individual studies have advocated twice weekly fetal surveillance starting from 32 weeks for all insulin treated GDM patients and reported a lower rate of stillbirth.[18] Intrapartum fetal monitoring includes regular and frequent auscultation of fetal heart and cardiotocography. Continuous fetal heart monitoring should be done wherever feasible.

FETAL BIOMETRY

From late second trimester to third trimester risk of many complications such as macrosomia, polyhydramnios, IUGR, and intrauterine fetal demise increases.[19] Macrosomia, which occurs in only 10% of nondiabetic pregnancies, complicates as high as 20–50% of pregnancies with diabetes. Abdominal circumference assessed at 28 weeks provides a clue about risk of macrosomia in index pregnancy while serial ultrasound scan provide a more accurate estimation of fetal weight.[20] Macrosomia is associated with significant perinatal and maternal morbidity and mortality in the form of shoulder dystocia, brachial plexus injury, birth trauma, perinatal mortality, and cesarean delivery. Polyhydramnios is also associated with high incidence of preterm labor, premature rupture of membranes, unstable lie, cord prolapse, and stillbirth.[21]

BIOPHYSICAL PROFILE

Role of BPP has not been studied in large populations of diabetic pregnancies but its proven value in other high-risk pregnancies can safely be applied in pregnancy complicated with diabetes too.[18] Twice weekly modified BPP is reported to be effective method of fetal assessment to prevent 1.4/1,000 stillbirths.[18]

INTRAUTERINE GROWTH RESTRICTION

Intrauterine growth restriction is not a common feature of pregnancy with diabetes. It is encountered in setting of placental insufficiency due to vasculopathy in long standing diabetes, comorbidities like preeclampsia, or due to overtreatment of GDM.[22] Sequential biometry with Doppler velocimetry of umbilical artery and middle cerebral artery has important role in monitoring such cases.

ROLE OF DOPPLER IN PREGNANCY COMPLICATED WITH DIABETES

Although American College of Obstetricians and Gynecologists and other guidelines recommend monitoring of diabetic pregnancy by Doppler velocimetry, but adverse fetal outcome which may be predicted with fair accuracy by Doppler of umbilical artery and middle cerebral artery in other high-risk pregnancies, fail to do, so in pregnancy with diabetes.[23,24] Cutoff values of impedance and other criteria of nondiabetic pregnancy cannot be applied to diabetic pregnancies. Even the diameter of the vessels is not same as other pregnancies. Doppler of ductus venosus and fetal hepatic arteries is found to be a better predictor of fetal compromise but its evaluation need further validation and expertise.

ASSESSMENT OF FETAL LUNG MATURITY

Pregnancies in diabetic women often need termination before term due to uncontrolled blood sugar, related comorbidities such as preeclampsia, deteriorating nephropathy, active proliferative nephropathy, and fetal compromise. Risk-benefit analysis is needed between continuation of pregnancy and respiratory distress syndrome (RDS) in baby due to delayed lung maturation. RDS is a major cause of neonatal morbidity and mortality in such pregnancies. Amniocentesis to assess the lecithin to sphingomyelin (L:S) ratio is a good option in borderline cases. If ratio is less than 2:1, prophylactic steroids are to be administered to accelerate lung maturity along with stringent blood sugar control to prevent hyperglycemia and ketoacidosis.[25] Ketoacidosis is a potential cause of fetal death in as high as 35% cases.[26] Maternal administration of steroid injection improves neonatal outcome, if preterm delivery between 23 weeks and 34 weeks of gestation is anticipated or planned. Routine administration of steroids for elective cesarean beyond 39 weeks is not recommended.

CONCLUSION

Pregnancies complicated with diabetes are at risk for increased fetal morbidity and mortality. Maintaining maternal plasma glucose levels within the euglycemic range in pregestational period and throughout the pregnancy and monitoring of fetus are the two essential elements of management of a diabetic pregnancy. Early first trimester scan for dating, early or second trimester aneuploidy screening,second trimester anomaly scan and fetal echocardiography should be offered to diabetic woman. Sequential growth scan and antenatal fetal testing should be done according to glycemic status and comorbidities of the patient.

KEY POINTS

- Maintaining maternal plasma glucose levels within the euglycemic range in pregestational period and throughout the pregnancy and monitoring of fetus are the two essential elements of management of a diabetic pregnancy.
- Early first trimester scan should be performed for correct dating of pregnancy.
- First trimester aneuploidy screening supported by ultrasonography targeted to nuchal translucency should be done.
- Second trimester aneuploidy screening followed by level II ultrasound scan should be offered at 18–20 weeks. Fetal echo may be done in high-risk cases.
- Base line biometry at 28 weeks followed by monitoring every 3–4 weekly for pregestational diabetes and type A2 GDM. Weekly fetal surveillance by NST, AFI, or BPP either alone or in combination is found to improve outcome. Frequency is increased to twice weekly towards term or in presence of obstetric complications.
- Diet controlled diabetes does not have increased risk of stillbirth and can be monitored by daily fetal movement count in cases of appropriate growth. Fetal surveillance may be applied according to local practice patterns towards term.

REFERENCES

1. DeSisto CL, Kim SY, Sharma AJ. Prevalence estimates of gestational diabetes mellitus in the United States, Pregnancy Risk Assessment Monitoring System (PRAMS), 2007–2010. Prev Chronic Dis. 2014;11:E104.
2. Raja MW, Baba TA, Hanga AJ, et al. A study to estimate the prevalence of gestational diabetes mellitus in an urban block of Kashmir valley (North India). Int J Med Sci Public Health. 2014;3:191-5.
3. Gopalakrishnan V, Singh R, Pradeep Y, et al. Evaluation of the prevalence of gestational diabetes mellitus in North Indians using the International Association of Diabetes and Pregnancy Study groups (IADPSG) criteria. J Postgrad Med. 2015;61(3):155-8.
4. Kayal A, Anjana RM, Mohan V. Gestational diabetes—An update from India. 2013. Diabetes Voice 58. 2013.
5. HAPO Study Cooperative Research Group, Metzger BE, Lowe LP, et al. Hyperglycemia and adverse pregnancy outcomes. N Engl J Med. 2008;358:1991-2002.
6. Becerra JE, Khoury MJ, Cordero JF, et al. Diabetes mellitus during pregnancy and the risks for specific birth defects: a population-based controlled study. Pediatrics. 1990;85:1-9.
7. Crowther CA, Hiller JE, Moss JR, et al. Effect of treatment of gestational diabetes mellitus on pregnancy outcomes. N Engl J Med. 2005;352(24):2477-86.
8. Dicker D, Feldberg D, Samuel N, et al. Spontaneous abortion in patients with IDDM: the effect of preconceptional diabetes control. Am J Obstet Gynecol. 1988;158:1161-4.
9. Fog Pedersen J, Molsted-Pedersen L. Ultrasound studies of fetal growth. In: Sutherland H, Stowers J, Pearson DWN (Eds). Carbohydrate Metabolism in Pregnancy and Newborn. Berlin: Springer-Verlag; 1989. pp. 83-93.

10. Sadler TW, Hunter ES III, Wynn RE, et al. Evidence for multifactorial origin of diabetes-induced embryopathies. Diabetes. 1989;38:70-4.
11. Savvidou M.D, Syngelaki A, Muhaisen M, et al. First trimester maternal serum free human chorionic gonadotropin and pregnancy-associated plasma protein A in pregnancies complicated by diabetes mellitus. BJOG. 2012;119:410–16.
12. Thornburg LL, Knight KM, Peterson CJ, et al. Maternal serum α-fetoprotein values in type 1 and type 2 diabetic patients. Am J Obstet Gynecol. 2008;199:e1-e5.
13. Bradley RJ, Brudenell JM, Nicolaides KH. Fetal acidosis and hyperlacticaemia diagnosed by cardocentesis in pregnancies complicated by maternal diabetes mellitus. Diabet Med. 1991;8:464-8.
14. Murthy EK, Renar IP, Metelko Z. Diabetes and pregnancy. Diabetologia Croatica. 2002;31(3):131-46.
15. Ben-Haroush A, Chen R, Hadar E, et al. Accuracy of a single fetal weight estimation at 29–34 weeks in diabetic pregnancies: Can it predict large-for-gestational-age infants at term? Am J Obstet Gynecol. 2007;197(5):497.e1-6.
16. Committee on Practice Bulletins—Obstetrics. Practice Bulletin No. 137: Gestational diabetes mellitus. Obstet Gynecol. 2013;122(2 Pt 1):406-16.
17. Committee on practice bulletins—Obstetrics Practice Bulletin No. 180: Gestational Diabetes Mellitus. Obstet Gynecol. 2017;130(1):e17-37.
18. Johnson JM, Lange IR, Harman CR, et al. Biophysical profile scoring in the management of the diabetic pregnancy. Obstet Gynecol. 1988;72:841-6.
19. Kc K, Shakya S, Zhang H. Gestational diabetes mellitus and macrosomia: a literature review. Ann Nutr Metab. 2015;66 Suppl 2:14-20.
20. Gilby JR, Williams MC, Spellacy WN. Fetal abdominal circumference measurements of 35 and 38 cm as predictors of macrosomia. J Reprod Med. 2000;45:936-8.
21. Idris N, Wong SF, Thomae M, et al. Influence of polyhydramnios on perinatal outcome in pregestational diabetic pregnancies. Ultrasound Obstet Gynecol. 2010;36:338-43.
22. American College of Obstetricians and Gynecologists Committee on Practice Bulletins—Obstetrics. ACOG Practice Bulletin. Clinical Management Guidelines for Obstetrician-Gynaecologists. Number 30, September 2001 (replaces Technical Bulletin Number 200, December 1994). Gestational diabetes. Obstet Gynecol. 2001:98(3):525-38.
23. Berger H, Gagnon R, Sermer M. Diabetes in Pregnancy. J Obstet Gynaecol Can. 2016; 38(7):667-79.e1.
24. Kiserud T. Diabetes in pregnancy: scanning the wrong horizon? Ultrasound Obstet Gynecol. 2010;36:266-7.
25. Piper JM, Langer O. Does maternal diabetes delay fetal pulmonary maturity? Am J Obstet Gynecol. 1993;168(3):783-6.
26. Bhagwanjee S, Muckart DJ, Hodgson RE, et al. Fatal outcome from diabetic ketoacidosis in pregnancy. Anaesth Intensive Care. 1995;23:234-7.

CHAPTER 19

Intrapartum Management of Diabetic Pregnancy

Chitra Sinha, Ritu Sharma

INTRODUCTION

Diabetes is a common medical condition complicating 6–9% of pregnancies. Ninety percent of the pregnant patients with diabetes will have gestational diabetes mellitus (GDM) and rest 10% will have pregestational diabetes mellitus (PGDM).[1,2] Among patients with GDM, 30–70% will have recurrence[3] and about 70% will develop diabetes 22–28 years after pregnancy.[4-6] Pregnancy with diabetes is a high-risk pregnancy because of the associated fetomaternal complications in antepartum, intrapartum, and postpartum periods. Complications in the intrapartum period include maternal complications [preterm labor, prolonged labor, increased operative interference, genital trauma, post partum hemorrhage (PPH) and sepsis]; and fetal complications (prematurity, shoulder dystocia, brachial plexus injury, stillbirth, respiratory distress, neonatal hypoglycemia, hypocalcemia, hyperbilirubinemia, and polycythemia).

TIMING AND MODE OF DELIVERY

The decision to deliver a patient with diabetes depends on maternal metabolic control, gestational age, and fetal growth assessment. There should be a balance between potential complications of stillbirth, macrosomia, and shoulder dystocia against the risk of premature delivery as well as potential complications of labor induction. Timing and mode of delivery should be discussed with the patient and their relatives in the antenatal period especially during third trimester. This will be helpful in future management.

Important Points Regarding Planning of Delivery

Timing and mode of delivery depends on type of diabetes, treatment received (diet, exercise, and pharmacological agents), and associated complications. Controlled GDM without any complications should not be delivered before 39 weeks unless indicated and pregnancy may be continued till 41 weeks. Complicated diabetes, i.e. uncontrolled diabetes in spite of hospitalization with aggressive efforts or abnormal fetal testing or associated complications like associated hypertension may need termination at less than 37 weeks

Table 19.1: Timing of delivery in pregnancy with diabetes.[7,8]

Diabetes in pregnancy	*Time of delivery (weeks)*
Controlled A1GDM (controlled on medical nutrition therapy)	39 to 40+6
Controlled A2GDM (controlled on pharmacotherapy)	39 to 39+6
Pregestational DM/poorly controlled GDM	37 to 38+6
Complicated diabetes	34 to 36+6

(GDM: Gestational diabetes mellitus).

of gestation. Pregnant women with type 1 or type 2 diabetes without other complications are advised to have an elective birth either by induction of labor, or by elective cesarean section, between 37 + 0 weeks and 38 + 6 weeks of pregnancy (Table 19.1).

If on ultrasound, macrosomic fetus is diagnosed, risk of vaginal delivery like shoulder dystocia brachial plexus injuries and PPH must be explained.[3] Mode of delivery—Diabetes is not a contraindication to vaginal birth. Lower segment cesarean section (LSCS) is indicated in case of estimated fetal weight more than or equal to 4.5 kg, bad obstetrical history, or any other obstetrical indication.

BLOOD GLUCOSE CONTROL DURING LABOR AND BIRTH

Goal of intrapartum management of diabetes in pregnancy is to maintain normoglycemia. Uncontrolled hyperglycemia in labor leads to fetal hyperinsulinemia and subsequently neonatal hypoglycemia. Fetal hyperglycemia and hyperinsulinemia also lead to increased fetal oxygen consumption resulting in fetal hypoxia and acidosis. The blood sugar target in labor recommended by various organizations varies between 70 mg/dL to 140 mg/dL (Table 19.2).

Insulin Requirement and Modes of Insulin Administration in Intrapartum Period

Requirement of insulin reduces significantly in active labor due to decreased hepatic gluconeogenesis and about eightfold increased calorie (glucose substrate) requirement. About 50% of the diabetic patients do not require insulin in active labor.[9,10] Patients with GDM controlled on diet do not require insulin, while patients with GDM on pharmacotherapy and pregestational diabetes may require low-dose insulin infusion in labor. Those requiring less than 20 U insulin per day usually do not need insulin in intrapartum period.

In those women who are on insulin, morning dose of insulin can be omitted. Capillary plasma glucose should be monitored every hour during active labor in women with diabetes. Insulin can be administered as

Table 19.2: Recommended blood sugar target in intrapartum period (mg/dL).

Organization	*Blood sugar (mg/dL)*
NIS, 2016	80–110
ACOG, 2013	70–110
CDA, 2013	72–126
RSSDI, 2016	70–140

(NIS: National Insulin Summit; ACOG: American College of Obstetricians and Gynecologists; CDA: Canadian Diabetic Association; RSSDI: Research Society for the Study of Diabetes in India).

Table 19.3: Insulin infusion in intrapartum period.

Blood glucose level (mg/dL)	*Insulin infusion (U/hour)*	*IV fluid*
<100	No	D5 RL
101–140	1	D5 RL
141–180	1.5	NS
181–220	2	NS
>220	2.5	NS

(IV: Intravenous; RL: Ringer's lactate; NS: Normal saline).

insulin infusion, neutralizing drip, intermittent subcutaneous insulin, and continuous subcutaneous insulin. Insulin infusion and intravenous fluids are to be given separately. The dose of insulin infused will depend on the blood glucose levels (Table 19.3).

Neutralizing drip can be made by adding fixed dose, usually 8 U of regular insulin or insulin analogs like insulin Lispro or insulin Aspart in 500 mL of 5% dextrose or dextrose normal saline (DNS) and giving it usually over 4 hours while maintaining the blood sugar targets. Intermittent subcutaneous insulin includes administration of 2–5 U of regular insulin in small doses at frequent intervals and this method is seldom practiced. Continuous subcutaneous insulin infusion is a probably the best method but the catheter is not freely available and is costly. So, mostly we are giving insulin either as infusion or as neutralizing drip.

OBSTETRIC MANAGEMENT

Usually the GDM patients go in spontaneous labor. Induction, if required should be planned ideally in the morning. Informed written consent is taken regarding the indication of induction, method of induction and the associated risks. The usual night dose of intermediate acting insulin is given. Fasting blood sugar, serum electrolytes and urine for sugar and ketones are sent in the morning. The morning dose of insulin is omitted. Capillary blood glucose monitoring is done hourly in active labor and insulin infusion is given accordingly.

Close monitoring of the labor events is essential to prevent maternal and fetal complication. Serum electrolytes and urine for sugar, ketones, and albumin should be evaluated every 4 hourly. Watch for any signs or symptoms suggestive of hypoglycemia or hyperglycemia. Progress of labor is to be monitored on partograph, so as to detect any abnormality at the earliest and intervene accordingly. Strict fetal heart rate monitoring is done preferably using CTG (cardiotocography). Per vaginal examinations are kept to the minimum to prevent sepsis. If due care has been given to asepsis and antisepsis, single dose prophylactic antibiotic will suffice. Liberal episiotomy is required to prevent genital trauma. One should be prepared to tackle shoulder dystocia, if encountered. Active management of third stage is important to prevent PPH. Placenta and umbilical cord should be monitored to detect any abnormalities. Care should be taken to avoid shoulder dystocia and brachial plexus injuries in cases of large for gestational age (LGA) fetuses.

Elective Cesarean Section

Patient is posted for cesarean section in morning as first case. The usual night dose of intermediate acting insulin is given but the morning dose is omitted. Fasting blood sugar, serum electrolytes, and urine for sugar and ketones are checked. If needed, start neutralizing drip or insulin and glucose infusion separately to maintain target blood glucose levels. Regional anesthesia is preferred as an awake patient can tell about the symptoms suggestive of hypoglycemia. Frequent blood sugar monitoring is required. If general anesthesia is given, monitor blood glucose every 30 minutes from induction till the woman is fully conscious.

Preterm Labor and Diabetes in Pregnancy

Fetal hyperglycemia and hyperinsulinemia interfere with the synthesis of surfactant and delays fetal lung maturity. Steroids should be administered in pregnant diabetic patient with preterm labor. After administration of steroids, the blood sugar levels begins to rise 12 hours after the first dose of steroid and the hyperglycemic effect lasts for 5 days. Therefore, frequent blood glucose monitoring is required as additional insulin may be required. Betamimetics should not be used as tocolytics, as they cause hyperglycemia. Magnesium sulfate is the drug of choice in these cases.

Neonatal Care

After delivery, the baby should be examined for any congenital malformations. Baby should be kept with the mother under observation for at least 24 hours. Breastfeeding should be initiated as early as possible preferably

Box 19.1: Indications for admission to neonatal intensive care unit (NICU).

- Hypoglycemia
- Hyperbilirubinemia
- Polycythemia
- Congenital heart disease
- Preterm baby (<34 weeks)
- Clinical signs
- Needs IV fluids

(IV: Intravenous).

within 30 minutes of birth and then continued every 2–3 hourly to maintain baby's blood glucose levels more than or equal to 47 mg/dL (>2 mmol/L) by frequent monitoring (2–4 hourly). If blood glucose levels are not maintained or the baby is not accepting orally or signs of hypoglycemia appear, start tube feeding or intravenous fluids. If there is appearance of abnormal clinical signs, send blood for various investigations like serum calcium, serum magnesium, bilirubin, and hematocrit. Echocardiography needs to be done, if there is suspicion of cardiomyopathy or congenital heart disease (Box 19.1).

IMMEDIATE POSTPARTUM CARE

Once the patient is delivered, the insulin requirement falls to half to two-third of the dose required in antenatal period due to loss of insulin resistance. So Insulin is stopped after delivery; blood glucose levels are done and insulin dose is adjusted accordingly.

CONCLUSION

Significant variation in the insulin requirement during labor and immediate postpartum period warrants strict blood sugar control, so as to have successful outcome of labor.

KEY POINTS

- Controlled GDM without any complications should not be delivered before 39 weeks unless indicated and pregnancy may be continued till 41 weeks.
- Complicated diabetes, i.e. uncontrolled diabetes in spite of hospitalization with aggressive efforts or abnormal fetal testing or associated complications like associated hypertension may need termination at less than 37 weeks.
- Pregnant women with type 1 or type 2 diabetes without other complications are advised to have an elective birth either by induction of labor, or by elective cesarean section, between 37 + 0 weeks and 38 + 6 weeks of pregnancy.

lipolysis, decreases glucose utilization, and increases maternal blood glucose levels. This action of HCS increases availability of glucose for fetus.

EFFECT OF MATERNAL DIABETIC ENVIRONMENT

Increased maternal blood glucose moves down the concentration gradient by facilitated diffusion from mother to fetus across the placenta. The placental endothelium expresses high affinity glucose transporter 1 (GLUT1) and GLUT3. The high level of glucose in fetus stimulates fetal pancreas beta cell mass to secrete more insulin which promotes fetal growth in diabetics (*Pedersen hypothesis—hyperglycemic-hyperinsulinism*).

EFFECTS OF FETAL HYPERINSULINEMIA

Fetal hyperinsulinemia leads to fetal macrosomia, fetal, and neonatal complications in diabetics and decreases the production of surfactant. This may occur through insulin receptors or through increased activity of insulin-like growth factor-1. The placental endothelium has insulin sensitive GLUT4. In the endothelium, insulin activates protein kinase B/Akt pathway,[1] alters gene expression,[2] and leads to increased glycogen synthesis.[3,4]

Fetal insulin also has indirect effects as a result of fetal hypoxia. Fetal insulin stimulates aerobic glucose metabolism and hence oxygen demand increases. Fetal hypoxia occurs as a result of decreased oxygen delivery and decreased uteroplacental blood flow.[5,6] Hypoxia stimulates angiogenesis,[7,8] hypercapillarization leading to increased placental weight and increased surface area for oxygen exchange in diabetics. Also, hypoxia leads to increased production of erythropoietin (EPA), leptin (LEP), adiponectin (ADIPOQ), placental growth factor (PlGF), angiopoietins (ANGPT), insulin/insulin-like growth factor (INS/IGF), vascular endothelial growth factor (VEGF), and fibroblast growth factor 2 (FGF2) which stimulate angiogenesis (Box 20.1).[9]

The diabetic placenta shows increase in diameter, central thickness, and weight. On histological examination, diabetic placentas showed increased number of villous capillaries and dilated blood vessels, villous edema, fibrinoid

Box 20.1: Mechanism for hypervascularity of placenta in diabetes: relation between glucose, oxygen and insulin.
Maternal hyperglycemia → Fetal hyperglycemia → Fetal hyperinsulinemia → Fetal macrosomia → Hypoxia → ↑EPA, LEP, ADIPOQ, PGF, ANGPT, IGF, VEGF, FGF → Placental angiogenesis
Hyperglycemia → Oxidative stress → Reactive oxygen species (ROS) → Proinflammatory cytokines like TNF-alpha, IL-6 →Placental angiogenesis

(EPA: Erythropoietin; LEP: Leptin; ADIPOQ: Adiponectin; PGF: Placental growth factor; ANGPT: Angiopoietins; IGF: Insulin-like growth factor; VEGF: Vascular endothelial growth factor; FGF: Fibroblast growth factor; TNF: Tumor necrosis factor; IL-6: Interleukin-6).

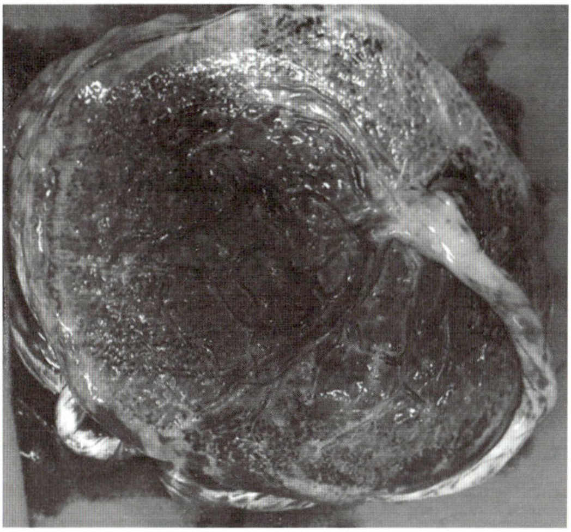

Fig. 20.1: Gestational diabetes mellitus (GDM) placenta. *(for color version see Plate 4)*

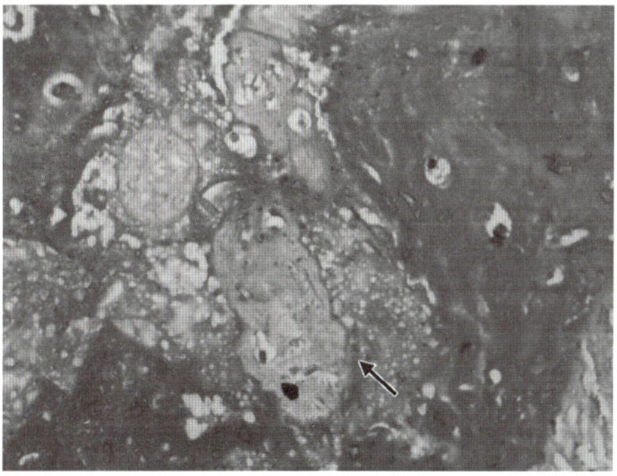

Fig. 20.2: Necrosed villi. *(for color version see Plate 4)*

deposits both extravillous and intravillous, thickening of the basement membrane of syncytiotrophoblast, glycogen deposits, increased interstitial collagen between the villous, and presence of fibrin and fibrosis in chorionic villi (Figs. 20.1 and 20.2).

PLACENTAL CYTOKINES

The human placenta synthesizes a variety of cytokines which regulate insulin action[9] in response to hyperglycemia. It includes tumor necrosis factor (TNF), leptin, and interleukin-6 (IL-6).

The trophoblast cells of placenta secrete leptin which acts on hypothalamus to regulate appetite, decrease food intake, and increases consumption of energy. There exists a feedback loop by which fasting decreases plasma leptin values and increased food intake, obesity increases leptin synthesis. Both endothelial cells and trophoblast express IL-6.[10] There is overexpression of these cytokines and hence enhanced insulin resistance in diabetes.[11-13]

ANTIDIABETIC AGENTS AND PLACENTA

Maternal insulin cannot pass through the placenta except with antibodies. Metformin has been shown to pass freely across the placenta while maternal-to-fetal transport of glyburide is significantly low or negligible.

CONCLUSION

Placenta is an important and dynamic link between the mother and the fetus and reflects the metabolic alterations of diabetic pregnancy.

KEY POINTS

- Increased maternal blood glucose moves down the concentration gradient by facilitated diffusion from mother to fetus across the placenta. The placental endothelium expresses high affinity glucose transporter 1 (GLUT1) and GLUT3. The high level of glucose in fetus stimulates fetal pancreas beta cell mass to secrete more insulin which promotes fetal growth in diabetics (Pedersen hypothesis—hyperglycemic-hyperinsulinism).
- Hyperglycemia increases oxidative stress and stimulates angiogenesis in the placenta.
- The diabetic placenta shows increase in diameter, central thickness, and weight.
- On histological examination, diabetic placentas showed increased number of villous capillaries and dilated blood vessels, villous edema, fibrinoid necrosis.
- Maternal insulin cannot pass through the placenta except with antibodies.
- Metformin has been shown to pass freely across the placenta while maternal to fetal transport of glyburide is significantly low or negligible.

REFERENCES

1. Hiden U, Maier A, Ghaffari-Tabrizi N, et al. Differential insulin receptor expression causes differential insulin signalling in the two interfaces of the human placenta. Placenta. 2005;26:A9.
2. Hiden U, Maier A, Bilban M, et al. Insulin control of placental gene expression shifts from mother to foetus over the course of pregnancy. Diabetologia. 2006;49:123-31.
3. Desoye G, Korgun ET, Ghaffari-Tabrizi N, et al. Selective upregulation of placental glycogenin-2 in gestational diabetes is independent of hyperglycemia or hyperinsulinemia. J Soc Gyn Invest. 2004;11 (Supp l.):299A.
4. Hahn D, Blaschitz A, Korgun ET, et al. From maternal glucose to fetal glycogen: expression of key regulators in the human placenta. Mol Hum Reprod. 2001;7:1173-8.

5. Fadda GM, D'Antona D, Ambrosini G, et al. Placental and fetal pulsatility indices in gestational diabetes mellitus. J Reprod Med. 2001;46:365-70.
6. Saldeen P, Olofsson P, Laurini RN. Structural, functional and circulatory placental changes associated with impaired glucose metabolism. Eur J Obstet Gynecol Reprod Biol. 2002;105:136-42.
7. Grosfeld A, Turban S, Andre J, et al. Transcriptional effect of hypoxia on placental leptin. FEBS Lett. 2001;502:122-6.
8. Lolmede K, Durand de Saint Front V, Galitzky J, et al. Effects of hypoxia on the expression of proangiogenic factors in differentiated 3T3-F442A adipocytes. Int J Obes Relat Metab Disord. 2003;27:1187-95.
9. Cvitic S, Desoye G, Hiden U. Glucose, Insulin, and Oxygen Interplay in Placental Hypervascularisation in Diabetes Mellitus. BioMed Res Int. 2014;145846.
10. Challier J, Galtier M, Bintein T, et al. Placental leptin receptor isoforms in normal and pathological pregnancies. Placenta. 2003;24:92-9.
11. Catalano PM, Hoegh M, Minium J, et al. Adiponectin in human pregnancy: implications for regulation of glucose and lipid metabolism. Diabetologia. 2006;49:1677-85.
12. Ranheim T, Haugen F, Staff AC, et al. Adiponectin is reduced in gestational diabetes mellitus in normal weight women. Acta Obstet Gynecol Scand. 2004;83:341-7.
13. Kinalski M, Telejko B, Kuzmicki M, et al. Tumor necrosis factor alpha system and plasma adiponectin concentration in women with gestational diabetes. Horm Metab Res. 2005;37:450-4.

CHAPTER 21

Infants of Diabetic Mother

Tanushree Sahoo, Ramesh Agarwal

INTRODUCTION

Diabetes is the most common metabolic disorder in pregnancy, which is associated with an increased maternal and neonatal morbidity.[1] Maternal diabetes may be pregestational (i.e. type 1 or type 2 diabetes diagnosed before pregnancy) or gestational (i.e. diabetes recognized during pregnancy). Perinatal outcome depends on the onset and duration of glucose intolerance and severity of the disease. Approximately 6–7% of all pregnancies are affected by abnormal glucose regulation out of which 90% are of gestational diabetes mellitus (GDM) while 10% are suffering from preexisting diabetes.[2,3] However, previous Indian studies have reported wide range of prevalence of GDM from as low as 3% to as high as 40%.[4-6] Infants of diabetic mothers (IDMs) possess significant medical problems, which are discussed here.

BACKGROUND AND PATHOPHYSIOLOGY

Till now no single pathogenic mechanism has been clearly defined to explain the various problems observed in IDMs. The most convincing Pedersen's hypothesis states that maternal hyperglycemia leads to fetal hyperglycemia, which in turn leads to fetal hyperinsulinism (Flowchart 21.1). Fetal hyperinsulinism leads to fetal hyperanabolism which is responsible for most of the morbidities.[7] In pregestational diabetes, uncontrolled hyperglycemia in the mother during fetal organogenesis may cause increased likelihood of fetal anomalies (fetopathy). In GDM, as the glucose intolerance occurs beyond the period of organogenesis, the risk of malformation remains unaltered. However, as the fetus is subjected to hyperglycemia in 2nd and 3rd trimester (embryopathy), due to transplacental passage of glucose, there is beta cell hypertrophy causing increased insulin production and consequent increased metabolism in the fetus. Being an anabolic hormone, insulin affects tissues such as adipocytes, skeletal and cardiac muscle, hepatic and connective tissue but not brain. It causes macrosomia without matching increase in head size resulting in shoulder dystocia during vaginal delivery.

Flowchart 21.1: Pathophysiology of infants of diabetic mothers.

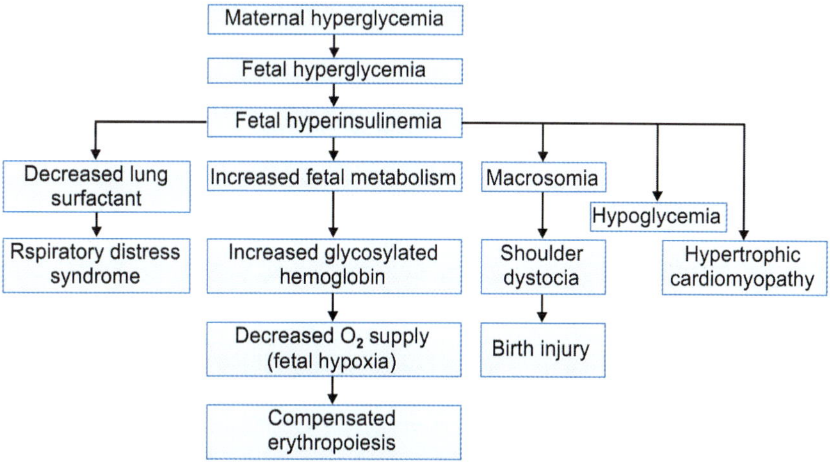

Table 21.1: Common malformations in infants of diabetic mothers.

System	*Malformation*
Cardiovascular	Transposition of great arteries, ventricular septal defect, coarctation, atrial septal defect, hypoplastic left heart, pulmonary stenosis, double outlet right ventricle, truncus arteriosus
Neurological	Anencephaly, microcephaly, holoprosencephaly, spina bifida
Gastrointestinal	Duodenal atresia, imperforate anus, situs inversus, cleft palate, small left colon syndrome
Musculoskeletal	Caudal regression or sacral agenesis, hemivertebrae, flexion contracture
Genitourinary	Urethral duplication, renal agenesis, hydronephrosis

PROBLEMS IN INFANTS OF DIABETIC MOTHERS

- *Congenital anomalies:* Incidence of congenital anomaly is 6–12% among IDMs born to women with pregestational diabetes. It is a leading cause (50%) of perinatal mortality among IDMs.[8,9] GDM is not associated with an increased risk of anomalies due to reason cited above. Various anomalies that are commonly found in GDM are given in Table 21.1. Out of which transposition of great arteries (TGA), small left colon syndrome and caudal regression syndrome are more commonly associated with IDMs. Caudal regression syndrome consists of incomplete development of sacrum, lumbar vertebrae—it occurs 200 times more frequently in IDMs as compared to others. Small left colon syndrome is a transient anomaly with 5% incidence in IDMs. It presents with features of intestinal obstruction and thus mimics Hirschsprung disease. Disturbance in

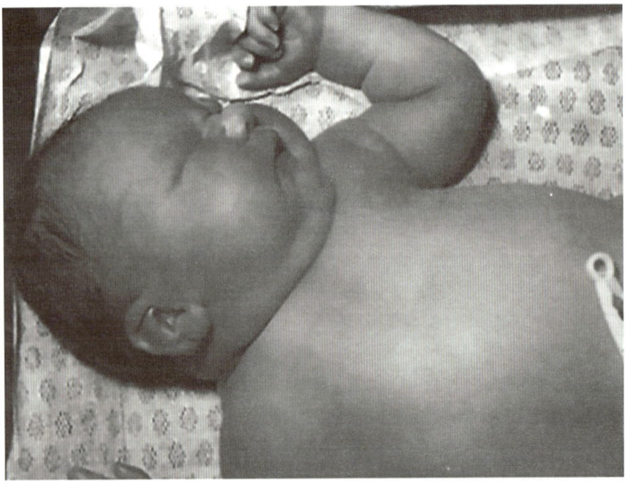

Fig. 21.1: Typical clinical feature of an infant of diabetic mother (note cherubic and suffused appearance with broad shoulders and upper trunk).*(for color version see Plate 4)*

autonomic nervous system is proposed as a cause. Strategy to reduce risk of congenital anomalies include preconceptional glycemic control (HbA1C level preferably below 7%) and intake of folic acid in periconceptional period.

- *Macrosomia*: Neonatal macrosomia, defined as birthweight more than or equal to 4,000 grams is a hallmark of IDMs, which results from insulin dependent increase in adiposity, and skeletal mass and liver mass. It happens towards midtrimester (20 to 30 weeks). Brain growth and head growth are usually spared. Therefore, there is disproportion between head and shoulder size as well as head and abdominal circumference. Macrosomia increases risk of shoulder dystocia and traumatic delivery (e.g. brachial plexus palsy, fracture of clavicle) and asphyxia.
- *Clinical features:* Typically, these infants appear large, chubby, suffused (due to polycythemia). They have relatively small head as compared to trunk, broad shoulder, and hairy pinna (Fig. 21.1).
- *Intrauterine growth retardation:* Occurs usually with severe pregestational diabetes (chronic hypertension, vascular disease) due to prolonged vascular insufficiency.
- *Hypoglycemia*: It is common and occurs both in large-for-gestational age (LGA), small-for-gestational age (SGA) IDMs. It usually happens shortly following delivery (30 to 90 min) and is due to abrupt cessation of maternally derived glucose after cord clamping while elevated insulin level continue to persist. However, this hyperinsulinemic state is self-limiting and resolve in 2–3 days. IDMs are less symptomatic (than non-IDMs), even with significant hypoglycemia.

- *Polycythemia*: IDMs often have polycythemia [defined as packed cell volume (PCV) more than 65%] as well as hyperviscosity syndrome. Possible explanations are increased erythropoietin production due to chronic fetal hypoxemia.[10,11] Because of hyperviscosity, they are predisposed to major vessel thrombosis (renal vein thrombosis) and tissue ischemia.
- *Hypocalcemia*: It is defined as total serum calcium of less than 7 mg/dL (1.8 mmol/L) or ionized calcium of less than 4 mg/dL (1 mmol/L) in IDMs may be asymptomatic or can have symptoms like jitteriness, seizures. Delay in surge of parathyroid hormone is possible hypothesis. Occurs usually 2–3 day after birth.[12]
- *Hypomagnesemia*: Defined as serum magnesium concentration less than 1.5 mg/dL (0.75 mmol/L) which can happen in up to 40% of IDMs and is postulated to be due to maternal hypomagnesemia secondary to increased urinary loss and prematurity. It is usually transient and does not require any treatment. However, if it is associated with hypocalcemia, then hypocalcemia may not respond to treatment unless hypomagnesemia is treated.[13,14]
- *Respiratory distress syndrome:* There is restriction of availability of substrate for surfactant protein synthesis due to hyperinsulinemic state as well as impaired type 2 pneumocyte function resulting in increased risk of respiratory distress syndrome up to 6-fold.[12,15] Similarly, due to fetal macrosomia, there is often inaccurate antenatal gestational assessment which often results inadvertent preterm delivery. Other causes of respiratory distress in IDMs include transient tachypnea of newborn (TTN) and cardiomyopathy.
- *Cardiomyopathy*: Various cardiomyopathy occurs in IDMs out of which asymmetric septal hypertrophy is most common.[16] It includes thickening of interventricular septum along with reduction in ventricular size. Most infants are asymptomatic although sometimes aortic outflow obstruction is severe enough to cause left ventricular failure. Hypertrophy is believed to be due to fetal hyperinsulinemia resulting in stimulation of cardiac muscle growth. Hypertrophy gradually resolves by age 6–12 months.[17] Symptomatic infants require supportive care in the form of fluid restriction and propranolol. Digitalis therapy can worsen the cardiac failure and is contraindicated.
- *Hyperbilirubinemia*: It is commonly found in IDMs which is supposed to be due to higher red cell mass, increased proportion of bruises secondary to macrosomia and increased red blood cell hemolysis.[13,18]
- *Decreased iron store:* The combined pool of storage iron and erythrocyte are lower in IDM which is secondary to shunting of iron to increased red cell mass. It is believed that relative low iron store can result in poor neurodevelopmental outcome later.

Table 21.2: Incidence of morbidities in infant of diabetic mothers.

Morbidities among infants of diabetic mothers (IDMs)	*Ohio, USA, 1998*[12]	*Thiruvananthapuram, India, 2012*[19]	*AIIMS, India, 2017*[20]
Large-for-gestational age	36%	-	29%
Macrosomia	-	3.4%	1%
Respiratory distress	34%	8.8%	11.2%
Hypoglycemia (symptomatic)	3.3%	7.5%	5.1%
Feeding problem	-	-	20%
Hyperbilirubinemia (Requiring phototherapy)	24%	-	10.2%
Polycythemia (Symptomatic)	5%	-	2%
Congenital malformation	5%	6.5%	0.5%

Along with good antenatal control of hyperglycemia as well as prompt postnatal management, incidences of various complications, especially of congenital malformation in IDMs, are decreasing over the year. Table 21.2 stated below depicts the same in form of a comparative data containing three studies (older study from 1998,[12] study from south India 2012[19] and a recent study done from author's institute 2017[20]).

MANAGEMENT

The current chapter mainly concentrates on postnatal management in IDMs. Major goal of management is anticipation and prompt management of any complication, if at all it arises.

- *DR preparation*: IDMs are more prone to have obstructed labor, birth asphyxia and birth trauma due to associated macrosomia. Hence attending neonatology team (consists of at least two doctors trained in Neonatal Resuscitation Program) should be anticipating this and be competent enough to handle all complications. Equipment for neonatal resuscitation should be pre-checked and kept ready in prior at resuscitation trolley.
- *Immediate postnatal management*
  - If cyanosis is detected, a detail cardiac evaluation followed by echocardiography is warranted.
  - Babies with respiratory distress should undergo clinical evaluation followed by chest radiogram to look for cardiomegaly and features of respiratory distress syndrome. Accordingly, respiratory support in form of continuous positive airway pressure and surfactant administration should be performed.

- *Breastfeeding challenges*:
    - Feeding problems are common among these infants due to macrosomia as well as higher rates of C-section. Thus, establishing early breastfeeding is of paramount importance and helps in preventing hypoglycemia.
- *Management thereafter*
    - Screening of all GDM for hypoglycemia as per the existing unit protocol. In authors' unit, first glucose monitoring is performed at 1–2 hours of birth. Subsequently, it is done at 6 hours, 12 hours, 24 hours and 48 hours of age.
- *Asymptomatic hypoglycemia*: If initial blood glucose value is less than or equal to 40 mg/dL and baby is asymptomatic, then an initial trial of supervised breastfeeding or paladai feeding is given. However, in case initial blood glucose value is less than or equal to 20 mg/dL or repeat blood glucose less than or equal to 40 mg/dL even after supervised feeding or palady feeding, intravenous (IV) glucose therapy is initiated. Initial starting glucose infusion rate (GIR) is 6 mg/kg/min, which are titrated depending on frequent blood glucose monitoring to maximum of 12 mg/kg/min.
- *Symptomatic hypoglycemia*: For all cases of symptomatic hypoglycemia, i.e. blood glucose value of less than or equal to 40 mg/kg with symptoms like jitteriness, lethargy, seizure. 200 mg/kg glucose is given as IV bolus and subsequently GIR is started similar to protocol for asymptomatic hypoglycemia.[21]
    - All neonates are screened for polycythemia by doing venous or capillary PCV at 2 hours of age and 6 hourly thereafter, if initial PCV is more than or equal to 65 till value is normalized. All symptomatic neonates in form of feed intolerance, jitteriness, hypoglycemia with PCV of more than or equal to 65, and any asymptomatic infant with PCV of more than or equal to 75 are managed with partial exchange.[21]
    - Routine measurement of calcium, magnesium and bilirubin is not required unless symptomatic.
    - If caudal dysplasia is suspected then detailed orthopedics evaluation should be done for ruling out involvement of femur, tibia, fibula and flexion contracture of knee and hip.
- Long-term outcomes:
    - *Catch down:* Infants of diabetic mothers due to effect of maternal hyperglycemia are often born with higher birthweight and length. However, it has been seen that these large-for-dates (LFD) babies often show catch down in growth in early childhood period typically between 6 months to 2 years of age, so that they ultimately grow in their own genetically determined trajectory[22,23] and achieve final growth comparable to their nondiabetic counterpart.

- *Metabolic syndrome*: There is gathering evidence that women with previous history of gestational diabetes are at increased risk of developing type 2 diabetes and cardiovascular disease in later age. Their adult offspring also has increased probability of developing components of metabolic syndromes like overweight or obesity, insulin resistance, higher blood pressure, renal disease, and type 2 diabetes. Factors like intrauterine hyperglycemia, genetics and environment may contribute to the pathogenesis.[24]

- *Neurodevelopment*: Uncontrolled maternal hyperglycemia during pregnancy is known to result in adverse neurodevelopmental outcome in offspring like low intelligence score, low intelligent quotient, short attention span and motor delay.[25,26]

CONCLUSION

Optimal management of IDMs require coordination between neonatologist and obstetrician in antenatal period followed by appropriate neonatal resuscitation. Prompt evaluation of anticipated complication helps in timely management of these babies and avoids unnecessary intervention. Long-term follow-up with particular concern for neurodevelopmental outcome and nutritional assessment is mandated.

REFERENCES

1. Landon M, Catalano P, Gabbe S. Diabetes mellitus complicating pregnancy. In: Gabbe SG, Niebyl JR, Galan HL, Jauniaux ERM, Landon MB, Simpson JL, Driscoll DA (Eds). Obstetrics: Normal and Problem Pregnancies. Philadelphia, PA: Churchill Livingstone/Elsevier; 2007. pp. 887-91.
2. Moyer VA, US Preventive Services Task Force. Screening for gestational diabetes mellitus: US Preventive Services Task Force recommendation statement. Ann Intern Med. 2014;160(6):414-20.
3. Committee on Practice Bulletins--Obstetrics. Practice Bulletin No. 137: Gestational diabetes mellitus. Obstet Gynecol. 2013;122(2 Pt 1):406-16.
4. Kalra P, Kachhwaha CP, Singh HV. Prevalence of gestational diabetes mellitus and its outcome in western Rajasthan. Indian J Endocrinol Metab. 2013;17(4):677-80.
5. Mithal A, Bansal B, Kalra S. Gestational diabetes in India: science and society. Indian J Endocrinol Metab. 2015;19(6):701-4.
6. Rajput R, Yadav Y, Nanda S, et al. Prevalence of gestational diabetes mellitus and associated risk factors at a tertiary care hospital in Haryana. Indian J Med Res. 2013;137(4):728-33.
7. Pedersen J. The Pregnant Diabetic and Her Newborn, 2nd edition. Baltimore: Williams and Wilkins; 1977.
8. Kitzmiller JL, Buchanan TA, Kjos S, et al. Pre-conception care of diabetes, congenital malformations, and spontaneous abortions. Diabetes Care. 1996;19(5):514-41.
9. Weintrob N, Karp M, Hod M. Short- and long-range complications in offspring of diabetic mothers. J Diabetes Complications. 1996;10(5):294-301.
10. Widness JA, Teramo KA, Clemons GK, et al. Temporal response of immunoreactive erythropoietin to acute hypoxemia in fetal sheep. Pediatr Res. 1986;20(1):15-9.

11. Widness JA, Teramo KA, Clemons GK, et al. Direct relationship of antepartum glucose control and fetal erythropoietin in human type 1 (insulin-dependent) diabetic pregnancy. Diabetologia. 1990;33(6):378-83.
12. Cordero L, Treuer SH, Landon MB, et al. Management of infants of diabetic mothers. Arch Pediatr Adolesc Med. 1998;152(3):249-54.
13. Rosenn B, Miodovnik M, Tsang R. Common clinical manifestations of maternal diabetes in newborn infants: implications for the practicing pediatrician. Pediatr Ann. 1996;25(4):215-22.
14. Banerjee S, Mimouni FB, Mehta R, et al. Lower whole blood ionized magnesium concentrations in hypocalcemic infants of gestational diabetic mothers. Magnes Res. 2003;16(2):127-30.
15. Robert MF, Neff RK, Hubbell JP, et al. Association between maternal diabetes and the respiratory-distress syndrome in the newborn. N Engl J Med. 1976;294(7):357-60.
16. Georgieff MK, Landon MB, Mills MM, et al. Abnormal iron distribution in infants of diabetic mothers: spectrum and maternal antecedents. J Pediatr. 1990;117(3):455-61.
17. Way GL, Wolfe RR, Eshaghpour E, et al. The natural history of hypertrophic cardiomyopathy in infants of diabetic mothers. J Pediatr. 1979;95(6):1020-5.
18. Peevy KJ, Landaw SA, Gross SJ. Hyperbilirubinemia in infants of diabetic mothers. Pediatrics. 1980;66(3):417-9.
19. Bhat M, Ramesha KN, Sarma SP, et al. Outcome of gestational diabetes mellitus from a tertiary referral center in South India: a case-control study. J Obstet Gynaecol India. 2012;62(6):644-9.
20. Wazid A, Deorari AK, Agarwal R, et al. Short term outcomes in term and late preterm neonates born to mothers with gestational diabetes. New Delhi: All India Institute of Medical Sciences; 2017.
21. Agarwal R, Deorari A, Paul VK. AIIMS Protocols in Neonatology, 1st edition. New Delhi: CBS Publishers and Distributors; 2015.
22. Touger L, Looker HC, Krakoff J, et al. Early growth in offspring of diabetic mothers. Diabetes Care. 2005;28(3):585-9.
23. Chiavaroli V, Cutfield WS, Derraik JGB, et al. Infants born large-for-gestational-age display slower growth in early infancy, but no epigenetic changes at birth. Sci Rep. 2015;5:14540.
24. Clausen TD, Mathiesen ER, Hansen T, et al. Overweight and the metabolic syndrome in adult offspring of women with diet-treated gestational diabetes mellitus or type 1 diabetes. J Clin Endocrinol Metab. 2009;94(7):2464-70.
25. Adane AA, Mishra GD, Tooth LR. Diabetes in Pregnancy and Childhood Cognitive Development: A Systematic Review. Pediatrics. 2016;137(5).
26. Bytoft B, Knorr S, Vlachova Z, et al. Long-term Cognitive Implications of Intrauterine Hyperglycemia in Adolescent Offspring of Women with Type 1 Diabetes (the EPICOM Study). Diabetes Care. 2016;39(8):1356-63.

CHAPTER 22

Postpartum Management after GDM

Pikee Saxena, Poonam Gupta

INTRODUCTION

While the importance of antenatal screening for gestational diabetes mellitus (GDM) is well-recognized, postpartum follow-up is not given its due importance. Health professionals and women with GDM are not aware about the significance of postpartum care.

A woman with history of GDM is at increased risk for developing GDM in subsequent pregnancies. The magnitude of risk increases with history of repeated episodes of GDM. Approximately 33%–66% of women with GDM will develop GDM in a subsequent pregnancy. In a study including 78,228 pregnancies the risk of GDM in women with and without previous GDM was 41% versus 4%. Chances of recurrence during second [OR, 13.2; 95% (confidence interval) CI 12.0–14.6) and third pregnancy (OR, 25.9; 95% CI 17.4–38.4] increase progressively.[1]

Besides recurrence of GDM, these women are more prone to develop type 2 diabetes mellitus DM (approximately 50% develop DM within 20 years), hypertension, dyslipidemia, metabolic syndrome and cardiovascular disease later in life.

Children exposed to hyperglycemia during pregnancy suffer from childhood obesity, impaired glucose tolerance and during adult life develop type 2 DM, metabolic syndrome and cardiovascular diseases.

Screening for hyperglycemia after delivery provides a unique opportunity to initiate healthy lifestyle practices or prophylactic medication to prevent or delay future development of diabetes. The US Diabetes Prevention Program (DDP) has provided evidence that lifestyle change reduce risk of developing Type 2 DM by 50%[2] and the effect of prevention of diabetes continued 10 years after lifestyle intervention.[2]

POSTPARTUM SCREENING FOR GLYCEMIC STATUS

The prevalence of prediabetes is seen in about 10%[3] of the women with GDM. Screening in the early postpartum period might detect hypo or hyperglycemia in the patients. There is a sudden reduction in insulin resistance after delivery of the placenta, resulting in improved insulin sensitivity and decreased insulin requirements. Increased metabolic demands of breastfeeding also reduce blood glucose and insulin requirement. After delivery of a woman with GDM, third day postpartum fasting and postprandial glucose levels should be monitored.

Women with GDM should discontinue blood glucose lowering therapy after delivery. Women with preexisting type 2 DM who are breastfeeding can resume metformin and glibenclamide therapy immediately after birth. Women with preexisting type 2 DM who were on insulin should reduce their insulin doses and monitor blood glucose levels carefully to establish appropriate dose.

It is recommended that GDM women should undergo fasting blood glucose (FBG) or 75 g, oral glucose tolerance test (OGTT) or HbA1c 4–6 months after delivery.In a follow-up study on 77 Asian Indian women, women with normoglycemia were 55, impaired fasting glucose (IFT) were 5, impaired glucose tolerance (IGT) were 9, combined impaired fasting glucose tolerance (IFT) and impaired glucose tolerance (IGT) were 8 and with Type 2 DM were 4.[3] Therefore, screening at 3 months postpartum may pick up substantial number of women with glucose abnormalities.

Various international authorities have recommended different tests and time duration to evaluate glycemic status after delivery (Table 22.1).

Interpretation of Postpartum Glucose Testing

- *Normal postpartum glucose test*: Fasting blood glucose (FBG) < 100 mg/dL and 2 hrs, 75 g < 140 mg/dL.
- *Overt DM*: Fasting blood glucose (FBG) ≥ 126 g/dL or 2 hrs 75 g ≥ 200 g/dL or HbA1c > 6.5%.

Table 22.1: Glucose screening tests recommended by various authorities.

Authority	*Recommended screening test*	*Timing of screening after delivery*
NICE (National Institute for Health and Clinical Excellence)[4]	Fasting glucose Fasting glucose/HbA1c	6–13 weeks After 13 weeks
Ministry of Health and family Welfare (MOHFW)[5]	75 g oral glucose tolerance test (OGTT)	6 weeks
ACOG (American College of Obstetrician and Gynecologist)[6]	(preferred) 75 g OGGT/ Fasting glucose levels	6–12 weeks
ADA (American Diabetes Association)[7,8]	Fasting glucose/OGTT	4–12 weeks

Despite the discrepancy among societies regarding the tests, there is general agreement in terms of the target glucose levels.

Supervised lifestyle modifications result in reduced weight retention in women with GDM which may indirectly contribute to reduced risk of metabolic derangements in future.[14,15] Healthy diets are associated with decreased risk of diabetes. Total daily caloric need should be calculated. Postpartum caloric requirement is 25 kcal/kg/day in nonbreastfeeding and 27–30 kcal/kg/day in breastfeeding women. To avoid maternal hypoglycemia, mother should be advised to have meal before feeding. Neonatal hypoglycemia may be avoided by breastfeeding within 30 minutes of birth then every 2–3 hourly on demand.

USE OF METFORMIN

Metformin, a biguanide compound, acts by reducing hepatic glucose output and by increasing insulin sensitivity. This results in decreased glucose level without any risk of either hypoglycemia or weight gain. Due to these effects of Metformin, it is seen as an ideal first-line treatment for people with Type 2 DM and also seen as a particularly attractive drug for preventing or delaying onset of Type 2 DM in women with prediabetes.[16]

BARRIERS AND CHALLENGES FACED FOR HEALTHY POSTPARTUM LIFESTYLE

Studies from countries like Australia, United States, and the Netherlands have investigated the different barriers to postpartum lifestyle among women with a history of GDM.[16-18] Lack of time and energy was a common barrier that surfaced in the studies. The lack of child care support was also seen to be a common challenge that was faced by several women. Emotional distress and the feeling of being unwell were also reported in most of the cases. Financial barriers and domestic responsibility also surfaced as one the reasons for neglected postpartum care.

Women desire and intend to maintain healthy lifestyle to prevent future diabetes but find the effort challenging. Self-efficacy and social support are important determinants in this regard.

Thus bringing about awareness regarding the adversities of GDM is the first step that needs to be taken. Routine screening and follow-ups need to take place regularly which become the major challenges.

KEY POINTS

- Women with gestational diabetic mellitus (GDM) after delivery have a high chance of recurrence of GDM in subsequent pregnancy and 50–60% lifetime risk of developing DM.
- All GDM women should undergo periodic 2 hrs 75 g OGTT screening at 6–12 weeks postpartum for detecting IFG IGT or DM. The test should be repeated after every 1–3 years.

- The importance of breastfeeding and effective family planning should be emphasized.
- Lifestyle modifications including healthy diet and exercise and pharmacotherapy to reduce the chronic disease risk should be adopted and followed to prevent or delay DM.
- Interconceptional counseling after GDM may prevent development of GDM in subsequent pregnancies and would reduce subsequent maternal and fetal complications associated with hyperglycemia in pregnancy.

REFERENCES

1. Getahun D, Fassett MJ, Jacobsen SJ, et al. Gestational diabetes: risk of recurrence in subsequent pregnancies. Am J Obstet Gynecol. 2010;203(5):467e1-6.
2. The Diabetes Prevention Program Research Group. The Diabetes Prevention Program: design and methods for a clinical trial in the prevention of type 2 diabetes. Diabetes Care. 1999;22(4):623-34.
3. Kitzmiller JL, Dang-Kilduff L, Taslimi MM. Gestational diabetes after delivery. Short-term management and long-term risks. Diabetes Care. 2007;30(2):225-35.
4. Diabetes in pregnancy: management from preconception to the postnatal period. NICE guideline [NG3]. 2015.
5. Sanjay Kalra, Yashdeep Gupta. Postpartum Screening of Gestational Diabetes: Opportunities for Integration with Existing Public Health. Indian J Community Med. 2015;40(3):209-10.
6. Knowler WC, Barrett-Connor E., The Diabetes Prevention Program Research Group. Reduction in the incidence of type 2 diabetes with lifestyle intervention or metformin. N Engl J Med. 2002;346(6):393-403.
7. ACOG Committee on Obstetric Practice. Postpartum screening for abnormal glucose tolerance in women who had gestational diabetes mellitus. Obstet Gynecol. 2009;113 (6):1419-21.
8. American Diabetes Association. Diagnosis and classification of Diabetes Mellitus. Diabetes Care. 2008;31:55-60.
9. Metzger B, Buchanan T, Coustan DR, et al. Summary and recommendations of the Fifth International Workshop—Conference on Gestational Diabetes Mellitus. Diabetes Care. 2007;30(2);251-60.
10. Karnik SK, Chen H, McLean GW, et al. Menin controls growth of pancreatic beta-cells in pregnant mice and promotes gestational diabetes mellitus. Science. 2007;318 (5851):806-9.
11. Kjos SL, Henry O, Lee RM, et al. The effects of lactation on glucose and lipid metabolism in women with recent gestational diabetes. Obstet Gynecol. 1993;82(3):451-5.
12. Crepaldi SC, Carneiro EM, Boschero AC. Long-term effect of prolactin treatment on glucose-induced insulin secretion in cultured neonatal rat islets. Horm Metab Res. 1997;29(5):220-4.
13. World Health Organization. (2015). Medical Eligibility Criteria for Contraceptive Use. [online] Available from http://www.who.int/reproductivehealth/publications/family planning/mec-wheel-5th/en/. [Accessed December 2017].
14. Alberti, KG, Zimmet PZ. Definition, diagnosis and classification of diabetes Mellitus and its complication. Part 1: diagnosis and classification of diabetes mellitus. Provisional report of a WHO Consultation. Diabet Med.1998;15(7):539-53.

15. Charle B, Norris R, Xiao X, et al. Population pharmacokinetics of metformin in late pregnancy. The Drug Monit. 2006;28(1):67-72
16. Rowan JA, Hague WM, Gao W, et al. Metformin versus insulin for the treatment of gestational diabetes. N Engl J Med. 2008;358(19):2003-15.
17. Niklas JM, Zera CA, England LJ. A web based lifestyle intervention for women with recent gestational diabetes mellitus: a randomized controlled trial. Obstet Gynecol. 2014;124(3):563-70.
18. Phelan S, Phipps MG, Abrams B. Does behavioural intervention in pregnancy reduce postpartum weight retention? Twelve-months outcomes of the Fit for Delivery randomized trial. Am J Clin Nutr. 2014;99(2):302-11.

CHAPTER 23

Benefits of Breastfeeding in Mothers with Gestational Diabetes

Pikee Saxena, Jyoti Gaur

INTRODUCTION

The prevalence of gestational diabetes mellitus (GDM) has increased by more than 30%[1,2] within last few decades and GDM has emerged as a worldwide epidemic. GDM is related to substantial short- and long-term adverse health outcomes. Although GDM commonly reverts back to normal glucose tolerance after pregnancy but the risk of developing type 2 diabetes mellitus (T2DM) later in life is 7 times higher in women with GDM than in women without it.[3] There are some unique problems associated with breastfeeding in diabetic mothers. Benefits of breastfeeding for the offspring have been known for long but the short- and long-term benefits for both the GDM mother and her child need to be highlighted. Breastfeeding delays the development of diabetes and metabolic syndrome for both by favorably influencing the carbohydrate and lipid metabolism.

REASONS FOR LOWER RATE OF BREASTFEEDING IN GESTATIONAL DIABETES MELLITUS

Several reasons have been proposed to explain the lower rate of breastfeeding in women with diabetes. Initiation of breastfeeding is more difficult for women with insulin-dependent diabetes and obese women due to physiologically lower levels of prolactin. There are higher rates of pregnancy and neonatal complications in women with GDM like prematurity, macrosomia, cesarean delivery due to fetopelvic disproportion and neonatal metabolic complications like hypothermia, hypocalcemia, hypoglycemia, polycythemia, and hyperbilirubinemia. These may delay the initiation of breastfeeding, deprive the neonate of the essential colostrum and may pose significant challenges to breastfeeding success. The rate of early breastfeeding was reported to be lower after cesarean section than after vaginal delivery,[4] which can be explained by above mentioned reasons.

MECHANISM INVOLVED IN LOWERING PLASMA GLUCOSE WHILE BREASTFEEDING

Epidemiologic studies suggest that breastfeeding reduces the risk of progression to T2DM after a GDM pregnancy by improving insulin resistance. The mammary gland expresses insulin receptors and is extremely sensitive to insulin during lactation. Therefore due to increased insulin sensitivity there is increased glucose disposal by the mammary gland. It has been indicated that circulating glucose could be preferentially diverted to the mammary gland via insulin-independent pathway to satisfy the demands of lactogenesis. This diversion may reduce the glucose load on pancreatic β cells and preserve long-term insulin production.[5]

Breastfeeding-related hormones, like prolactin, play an important role in improving glucose homeostasis by stimulating insulin secretion from pancreatic β cells islets.[6,7] Menin is a protein which has antiproliferative effects on β cells, leading to impaired glucose tolerance in the pregnant women. Prolactin causes downregulation of menin, in pregnant and lactating women.[7]

Formula feeding of babies is responsible for increasing the levels of hormones ghrelin which increases insulin secretion and body fat accumulation in formula-fed babies.[8]

LACTOGENESIS IN WOMEN WITH GESTATIONAL DIABETES MELLITUS

Maternal diabetes and obesity can delay the onset of lactogenesis in women with GDM. Milk feeding supplementation may also interfere with maternal milk production. In obese mothers, lactogenesis is impaired by lower physiological level of prolactin in response to suckling. Thus, among the obese women lower rates and short duration of breastfeeding is caused by delayed milk production. Women with GDM have more difficulty in expressing the colostrum from their breasts during the first 2 days of lactation.[9]

EFFECTS OF BREASTFEEDING ON MATERNAL METABOLIC PARAMETERS

It has been seen that prolonged breastfeeding is associated with 2 kg maternal weight loss by 1 year postpartum[10] as well as smaller waist circumference.[11] Longer duration of breastfeeding results in lower maternal weight gain after 10–15 years of postpartum.[12] The extra calories of 400–500 kcal/day required for milk production for first 6 months are derived from maternal dietary intake, additional 170 kcal/day come from the mobilization of fat stores.[4,13] About 50 g/day glucose is diverted for milk production through noninsulin-dependent pathways of uptake by mammary glands. Therefore, breastfeeding women have lower level of blood glucose and insulin concentration along with higher rates of glucose production and lipolysis.[14]

One cross-sectional study of Letinas et al. with previous GDM showed that women who breastfeed have lower total area under the glucose tolerance curve and lower fasting serum glucose after controlling for BMI, maternal age, and insulin use during pregnancy.[15]

Short-term Effects of Breastfeeding in Women with Gestational Diabetes Mellitus

A cross-sectional study which involved subsequent follow-up assessment after delivery was conducted by Kjos et al.[16] At the first follow-up visit at 4–12 weeks postpartum, glucose, and lipid metabolism were improved in the lactating group in terms of significantly lower total area under the curve (AUC) for glucose, lower mean fasting serum glucose, lower mean 2-h glucose, and higher mean serum high-density lipoprotein-cholesterol after adjusting for maternal age, BMI, and the use of insulin during pregnancy.[16] The two groups were matched for age, weight, weight loss by 3 months postpartum, and their exercise habits. At 3 months postpartum, insulin sensitivity, glucose responses, or adiposity (subcutaneous and visceral fat measured by computed tomography) were not significantly different between the two groups. However, the disposition index (DI), which was calculated as insulin sensitivity × acute insulin response to glucose, was significantly higher in breastfeeding women than in nonbreastfeeding women. Disposition index represents the ability of pancreatic β cells to compensate for insulin resistance. Thus, breastfeeding in mothers with GDM is associated with improved pancreatic β-cell function, for short term.[16]

Long-term Effects of Breastfeeding in Women with Gestational Diabetes Mellitus

A retrospective study evaluated the development of T2DM in GDM women during a follow-up of 20 years.[10] There were a few limitations of the study like lack of standardized oral glucose tolerance tests (OGTTs) at specific times after pregnancy, lack of detailed measures on breastfeeding (i.e. duration and intensity), self-report of GDM or T2DM diagnosis, recall bias regarding lactation duration, lack of control for confounders (e.g. physical activity and diet, differences in postpartum BMI). The authors observed that for every year, a woman who breastfed, has 15% less chances for the development of T2DM (Table 23.1). This protective effect appears to begin after 6 months of breastfeeding which is independent of maternal BMI and lifestyle behaviors (i.e. amount of exercise, diet, and smoking). However, breastfeeding had a clinically insignificant effect on the risk of T2DM among high-risk women with GDM, with a risk reduction of just 4%.[10] According to a German GDM meta-analysis study it has been found that breastfeeding is associated with the reduced risk of acute otitis media, nonspecific gastroenteritis, severe lower respiratory tract infections, atopic dermatitis, asthma, obesity, T1DM, T2DM, childhood leukemia, sudden infant death syndrome (SIDS), and necrotizing enterocolitis.[20] It helps to build a special relationship between mother and child, lowers the cost of artificial feed for the family and reduces the chances of infection.

The other benefits for the mother are that as breastfeeding inhibits ovulation it reduces exposure to estrogen and reduces incidence of breast and ovarian cancer, improves endometriosis and acts as an effective contraceptive method. These benefits reduce short- and long-term morbidity, mortality for the woman and the infant and also lower financial and psychological burden for the family and the nation.

CONCLUSION

Breastfeeding improves the glucose and lipid metabolism in women with GDM and also reduces the risk of T2DM. These women have lower maternal BMI, improved biochemical factors during reproductive years, lower incidence of metabolic disorders, breast cancer and ovarian cancer. Breastfeeding also provides a natural and effective means of contraception during the postpartum period. At 4–12 weeks postpartum, lactation is associated with improved glucose tolerance, fasting glucose, and total area under the glucose tolerance curve. The World Health Organization recommends exclusive breastfeeding for 6 months of age, and breastfeeding should be continued with appropriate complementary foods for 2 years or longer.[21,22]

KEY POINTS

- Breastfeeding has its long-term and short-term beneficial effects on GDM mother and her offspring.
- Women with GDM who breastfeed have a short-term lower level of blood sugar and lipid profile and it also helps to lose weight as extra calories are utilized in lactogenesis in a noninsulin-dependent manner.
- Breastfeeding for more than 3–6 months may delay or postpone the development of T2DM and metabolic syndrome by several years.
- Breastfeeding lowers blood sugar of the newborn in the neonatal period. Breastfed children have a lower risk of developing obesity, T2DM and metabolic syndrome in later life. It lowers the rates of diarrhea and respiratory tract infection.
- Exclusive breastfeeding acts as an effective contraceptive measure, helps in emotional bonding between the mother and her neonate and in the long run and reduces the risk of ovarian cancer and breast cancer.

REFERENCES

1. Anna V, van der Ploeg HP, Cheung NW, et al. Sociodemographic correlates of the increasing trend in prevalence of gestational diabetes mellitus in a large population of women between 1995 and 2005. Diabetes Care. 2008;31:2288-93.
2. Guariguata L, Linnenkamp U, Beagley J, et al. Global estimates of the prevalence of hyperglycaemia in pregnancy. Diabetes Res Clin Pract. 2014;103:176-85.
3. Bellamy L, Casas JP, Hingorani AD, et al. Type 2 diabetes mellitus after gestational diabetes: a systematic review and meta-analysis. Lancet. 2009;373:1773-9.
4. Butte NF, Hopkinson JM, Mehta N, et al. Adjustments in energy expenditure and substrate utilization during late pregnancy and lactation. Am J Clin Nutr. 1999;69:299-307.
5. Crepaldi SC, Carneiro EM, Boschero AC. Long-term effect of prolactin treatment on glucose-induced insulin secretion in cultured neonatal rat islets. Horm Metab Res. 1997;29:220-4.
6. Karnik SK, Chen H, McLean GW, et al. Menim controls growth of pancreatic beta-cells in pregnant mice and promotes gestational diabetes mellitus. Science. 2007;318: 806-9.
7. Stuebe AM, Rich-Edwards JW, Willett WC, et al. Duration of lactation and incidence of type 2 diabetes. J Am Med Assoc. 2005;294:2601-10.
8. Tschöp M, Smiley DL, Heiman ML. Ghrelin induces adiposity in rodents. Nature. 2000;407:908-13.
9. Rasmuseen KM, Kjolhede CL. Prepregnant overweight and obesity diminishes the prolactin response to suckling in the first week postpartum. Pediatrics. 2004;113: e465-e71.
10. Dewey KG, Heinig MJ, Nommsen LA. Maternal weight-loss patterns during prolonged lactation. Am J Clin Nutr. 1993;58:162-6.
11. Gigante DP, Victoria CG, Barros FC. Breast-feeding has a limited long-effect on anthropometry and body composition of Brazilian mothers. J Nutr. 2001;131:78-84.
12. Rooney BL, Schauberger CW. Excess pregnancy weight gain and long-term obesity: one decade later. Obstet Gynecol. 2002;100:245-52.
13. Stettler N, Srallings VA, Troxel AB, et al. Weight gain in the first week of life and overweight in adulthood: a cohort study of European American subjects fed infant formula. Circulation. 2005;111:1897-903.
14. Tigas S, Sunehag A, Haymond MW. Metabolic adaptation to feeding and fasting during lactation in humans. J Clin Endocrinol Metab. 2002;87:302-7.
15. Kjos SL, Henry O, Lee RM, et al. The effect of lactation on glucose and lipid metabolism in women with recent gestational diabetes. Obstet Gynecol. 1993;82:451-5.
16. Ziegler AG, Wallner M, Kaiser I, et al. Long-term protective effect of lactation on the development of type 2 diabetes in women with recent gestational diabetes mellitus. Diabetes. 2012;61:3167-71.
17. Chouinard-Castonguay S, Weisnagel JS, Tchernof A, et al. Relationship between lactation duration and insulin and glucose response among women with prior gestational diabetes. Eur J Endocrinol. 2013;168:515-23.
18. National Collaborating Centre for Women's and Children's Health. Diabetes in Pregnancy: Management of Diabetes and its Complication from Preconception to the Postnatal Period. London: RCOG Press; 2008.

should be made on the preference and individual risk factor of the particular woman. Choosing a safe and reliable method needs to make a reference to World Health Organization (WHO) medical eligibility criteria update 2015.

DIFFERENT METHODS OF CONTRACEPTION

Combined Hormonal Contraception

These methods include combined oral contraceptive (COC) pills, transdermal contraceptive patches, combined vaginal rings, and combined injectable contraception.

Combined hormonal contraception and its relation to carbohydrate metabolism: Older high dose combined hormonal pills resulted in impaired glucose tolerance test in many women. Plasma levels of insulin as well as glucose were elevated. Generally the effect of hormones is to produce an increase in peripheral resistance to insulin action. Most women can meet this challenge by increasing insulin secretion and there is no change in glucose tolerance test.

Insulin sensitivity is affected mainly by the progestin component. The derangement of carbohydrate metabolism may also be affected by estrogen influences on lipid metabolism, hepatic enzymes and elevation of unbound cortisol. Levonorgestrel has been associated with decreased insulin sensitivity. However, pills containing drospirenone, desogestrel, or gestodene tend to be metabolically neutral in terms of carbohydrate metabolism. But in recent years, with low dose of hormones, the results of Cochrane reviews of many RCTs have failed to detect any increase in the incidence of DM or impaired glucose tolerance. Data now strongly indicates that changes in carbohydrate metabolism are not clinically meaningful. The minor hyperglycemia is not deleterious and is completely reversible.[2]

Another study has found no evidence of vascular complications developing in young women with IDDM using hormonal pills.[3]

Combined Oral Contraceptive Pills

Combined oral contraceptive pills can safely be used by women with DM without vascular complications. However, they should be avoided in women with risk factors, such as above 35 years of age, smoking, obesity, migraine with aura, current breast cancer or history of breast cancer with active disease within 5 years, having DM for more than 20 years and in patients who have evidence of end organ damage due to increased risk of venous thromboembolism, myocardial infarction and stroke. All combination therapy contains a range of ethinyl estradiol doses and varying types of progestins which prevent pregnancy by blocking the LH surge and by thickening cervical mucus. These have only 0.3% failure rate with perfect use and about 8% with typical use in the first year. However, continuation rate of COC use declines gradually.

These pills are preferred by many women for some noncontraceptive benefits, such as improvement in acne, reduction in dysmenorrhea, decreasing menstrual flow and suppression of ovarian cysts.

There are a number of minor side-effects associated with these pills. However, if a patient experiences any of the following five symptoms (memorized as "A-C-H-E-S"), a doctor should immediately be consulted:

1. Abdomen pain
2. Chest pain
3. Headaches (very severe)
4. Eye problems which include blurry vision, doubled vision, and high tolerance to light
5. Swelling or aching in the limbs.

Transdermal Contraceptive Patch

It is a contraceptive skin patch that delivers 0.15 mg of progesterone and 20 μg of estrogen daily. It is changed once weekly for 3 weeks. It is then removed to allow for a 1 week withdrawal bleed before placing the next patch. In a clinical trial it has been seen that obese women had a greater failure rate.[4]

Combined Vaginal Ring

NuvaRing, containing etonogestrel, an active form of desogestrel together with ethinyl estradiol, is a transparent flexible ring. It is inserted into the upper vaginal area which delivers a small dose of estrogen and progesterone daily for a total duration of 4 weeks. The steroid hormones in the ring are absorbed directly through the vaginal mucosa minimizing first pass metabolism through the liver and causing 30–40% less hormone exposure than oral administration. The advantage is fewer side effects. It is an excellent method for women who prefer monthly administration and a method they can control themselves.

Combined Injectable Contraceptive

Injections have become a popular choice for women because of convenience and highly effective results. But side effects like bloating, weight gain, dizziness, unwanted hair growth, headache and anxiety episodes are there. After administration of the injection, patient will have to deal with the problem till the effects wear off.

Progesterone Only Pill

Progesterone only pill (POP) is regarded as a safe option for women with DM at any age with or without complication (WHO MEC 2). As this does not interfere with lactation, it is often chosen for breastfeeding women.

Along with optimization of insulin dosages before surgery, oral hypoglycemic agents should be stopped prior to surgery.

PERIOPERATIVE MANAGEMENT OF DIABETES

During perioperative period adequate blood sugar control is required to meet high energy requirements, without pushing the women toward hypoglycemia. Poor perioperative glycemic control increases the risk of neonatal hypoglycemia and increase in complications following surgery, especially nosocomial infection. Rise in blood glucose levels 4–6 hours before delivery can results in transient neonatal hypoglycemia.[13] Short and rapid-acting insulin can be used during labor to achieve normoglycemia.

GLYCEMIC TARGETS

Maternal hyperglycemia results in excessive secretion of insulin synthesis by the fetal pancreas, thereby increasing the risk of neonatal hypoglycemia. Thus, the National Institute of Clinical Excellence (NICE) 2015 recommends hourly capillary glucose monitoring during labor in women with diabetes, and maintaining a blood sugar between 70 mg/dL and 126 mg/dL (4–7 mmol/L).[13] An upper range of 110 mg/dL of capillary blood glucose (CBG) level during labor (6.1 mmol/L) has been recommended by the ACOG and the American College of Endocrinology.[14,15] The glycemic targets are same for type 1 DM, type 2 DM as well as gestational DM. A high risk of neonatal hypoglycemia (<31 mg/dL) has been associated with the maternal blood glucose value of more than 144 mg/dL during labor .[16]

INSULIN THERAPY IN PERIOPERATIVE PERIOD

During latent labor, hepatic glucose supply is adequate, but during active labor, hepatic glucose supply is restricted, therefore, further addition of calories is required. The supplementation is given by IV glucose, as the woman remains fasting in active labor.

The requirement of insulin during labor depends on the prior glycemic control during the antenatal period. Women with poor glycemic control during pregnancy need higher dose of insulin during labor both in active and latent labor. Women with good glucose control during pregnancy may not require very high dose of insulin during labor.

Insulin management of women with gestational diabetes mellitus (GDM), type 1 and type 2 DM is the same. Intravenous insulin infusion and dextrose infusion should be given for women with diabetes from onset of fasting with an aim of maintaining the CBG level within 70–126 mg/dL ((4–7 mmol/L). In the past, to reduce maternal hyperglycemia, the standard way of treatment was administration of insulin by the sliding scale subcutaneous regimen. But now, the recommended regimen is *variable rate IV insulin infusion.*[17] The

Table 25.1: Management of capillary blood glucose (CBG).

CBG	*Management*
<72 mg/dL (<4.0 mmol/L)	Stop the IV insulin infusion and consult physician
73–108 mg/dL (4.1–6.0 mmol/L)	Leave at the same insulin infusion rate
109–144 mg/dL (6.1–8.0 mmol/L)	Increase IV insulin infusion by 2 mL/hour
145–180 mg/dL (8.1–10 mmol/L)	Increase IV insulin infusion by 3 mL/hour
>180 mg/dL (>10 mmol/L)	Continue IV insulin infusion, seek medical advice

IV insulin infusion regimen is simple and has more predictable absorption compared with that of subcutaneous injection. Insulin infusion is prepared by dissolving 50 units of regular insulin in 50 mL of dextrose solution and started at the rate of 1 mL/hour. Dextrose infusion is formed by 10 mEq of KCl in 500 mL of 10% dextrose. Both dextrose and insulin are infused together in same IV line. CBG is measured hourly, and insulin or glucose infusion is adjusted according to Table 25.1.[18]

In clinical practice, 10 units of regular insulin is added to10% dextrose solution along with 10 mEq K^+ in the same solution and infusion is started at the rate of 100 mL/hour. However, if the need for insulin is high, a separate insulin infusion is preferred, with intensive monitoring of the blood glucose every 1-2 hours. Insulin infusion rates may be titrated accordingly and simultaneous glucose infusion may be started if the blood glucose falls.

MONITORING BLOOD SUGAR LEVELS

The rapid glucose metabolism during labor necessitates frequent CBG monitoring which should be 2–4 hourly in latent phase and 1–2 hourly in active phase. Measurement of CBG is generally an accurate method to check the blood glucose bedside except in extreme of ranges when values may not be reliable. Hence, laboratory confirmation of venous blood glucose may be required.

In women with GDM on diet, CBG should be monitored every 4-6 hours but in women with GDM on insulin, it is mandatory to do CBG 1-2 hourly in labor.

INTRAOPERATIVE MANAGEMENT

Interventional procedures like cervical cerclage, cystectomy, cesarean section (CS), induction of labor (IOL) or any other surgical procedures in diabetic mother induce physiological stress and release of counter regulatory hormones like cortisol, glucagon, which can induce hyperglycemia and a few can develop ketosis. The aim of monitoring in diabetic women is to avoid hyperglycemia and prevent ketoacidosis in mother.

CHAPTER 26

Bariatric Surgery and Gestational Diabetes: Implications

Aruna Nigam, Pikee Saxena

BURDEN OF OBESITY

The prevalence of obesity is increasing all over the world. According to World Health Organization (WHO) guidelines, body mass index (BMI) has been categorized into i.e. normal BMI (18.5–24.9 kg/m^2), overweight (25–29.9 kg/m^2), and obesity as a BMI more than or equal to 30 kg/m^2.[1] According to the WHO World Health Statistics Report 2012, globally one in six adults is obese and nearly 2.8 million individuals die each year due to overweight or obesity.[2] More than 36.5% adults in USA are obese and obesity is more prevalent among females (38.3%) as compared to men (34.3%).[3] Urban Indian data (female/male obesity prevalence is 31.3%/26.3%) is comparable to the USA. Thus, currently India is battling with both the problems of nutrition. As India battles the malnutrition mainly in rural area, the other problem of nutrition in the form of obesity is emerging in the urban area, and according to National Family Health Survey 2015-16 (NFHS-4), the prevalence of obesity has doubled up. Overall prevalence of obesity (BMI >25 kg/m^2) in India among women is 20.7%.[4] According to NFHS 4 in 2015–16 percentage of obese population is maximum in Delhi, Punjab, Tamil Nadu, Maharashtra, and Jharkhand. Obesity has significant negative impact on health by increasing rates of diabetes, hypertension, cardiovascular diseases, and degenerative joint disease. Moreover it has significant effect on economy by increasing the cost of medical care. The presence of obesity and metabolic syndrome in women of reproductive age is important because obesity is an independent risk factor for adverse maternal and neonatal outcomes and can lead to secondary diseases like type 2 diabetes (T2D) as well as gestational diabetes mellitus (GDM).

Incidence of bariatric surgery (BS) is increasing day by day because of increasing prevalence of obesity, easy laparoscopic access, financial availability, and concept of figure "0". In 2013–14 more than 6,500 BS were performed in females, out of which 78% were in females with more than half in the females of reproductive age group.[5] In the current chapter we will be discussing the implications of BS on pregnancy with regards to fetomaternal outcome.

PATHOPHYSIOLOGY OF EFFECT OF OBESITY ON DEVELOPMENT OF GESTATIONAL DIABETES MELLITUS

In a normal pregnancy, there is 60% reduction in the insulin sensitivity during pregnancy leading to development of GDM in many of these pregnant women. Presence of obesity further escalates the hyperglycemia of pregnancy because of preexistent baseline insulin resistance leading to higher chances of developing GDM in the obese females.[6] Thus, weight loss in obese females can improve the fetomaternal outcome by decreasing incidence of GDM and many other complications. Moreover future generation can also be prevented from the risk of developing obesity and diabetes as per the intrauterine long-term programmatic theory of obesity and diabetes.

Obesity is one of the most difficult health problem to deal. The weight loss in obese individual can be achieved by lifestyle modifications, drugs, diet control, and exercise, but these interventions are generally not successful because of ineffectiveness and weight regain. BS is a boon for the obese person as it provides sustainable and significant reduction in body weight (>60% excess weight loss), correction of comorbid conditions, and better survival.[7-9] Indications of BS in any individual are failure of trial of medical therapy and BMI more than 35 kg/m^2 with obesity-related comorbidities. Buchwald et al.[7,10,11] has shown that BS, especially gastric bypass, is an efficient means of managing and even curing T2D. This has created considerable interest in the efficacy of BS for preventing the development of GDM.

OVERVIEW OF BARIATRIC SURGERIES

There are several types of BS for the weight loss as described here.

Restrictive

These procedures achieve weight loss by reducing the food intake and also there is early and prolonged satiety after a solid meal. These include:

- *Laparoscopic adjustable gastric banding (LAGB):* Here the uppermost portion of the stomach is encircled by an inflatable balloon band which decreases the gastric volume. The diameter of this balloon can be altered by adding or removing saline as a day care procedure depending on the rate of a patient's weight loss.
- *Gastroplasty—laparoscopic sleeve resection (gastrectomy)/vertical band gastroplasty (VBG):* In this the upper part of the stomach is stapled to create a narrow gastric inlet or pouch which causes sense of fullness after eating small meals. VBG has now been superseded by adjustable band

procedures and procedures that combine mechanical restriction with bypass because of the poor long-term weight loss and complications.

Malabsorptive

Here certain length of small intestine is bypassed so that the food and digestive juices come in contact with only a short length of bowel causing malabsorption of the food and thus weight loss, i.e. jejunoileal bypass. These alone are not preferred these days.

Combined Restrictive and Malabsorptive

The procedures include:

- *Biliopancreatic diversion:* Here, 70% of the stomach is removed and a significant proportion of small intestine is bypassed which leads to malabsorption especially of fats caused by (1) diversion of food downstream and (2) reduction in the quantities of enzymes and bile in the bypassed segment.
- *Biliopancreatic diversion with duodenal switch:* This is rarely performed now due to substantial long-term complications of hepatic failure, renal failure, kidney stones, arthritis, and malnutrition.
- *Roux-en-Y gastric bypass (RYGB):* In this procedure, a part of stomach, whole of the duodenum, and 40–150 cm of the proximal jejunum are bypassed resulting in reduced absorptive area as well as changes in hormones [e.g. Ghrelin and peptide YY (PYY)] and neural signals to the gastrointestinal tract leading to hunger control and satiety. Patients generally develop an aversion to high-carbohydrate diet and make major changes in their diet and eating habits.

FETOMATERNAL COMPLICATIONS OF MATERNAL OBESITY

Maternal obesity increases the risk of miscarriages, hypertension, GDM, labor induction, cesarean delivery, postpartum hemorrhage, infectious morbidity, and thromboembolic events. Fetal risks include more chances of still birth, increased risk of birth defects, prematurity, macrosomia, birth trauma, and childhood obesity.

Table 26.1 delineates the effects of BS on occurrence of various fetomaternal complications.

EFFECT ON DEVELOPMENT OF GESTATIONAL DIABETES MELLITUS

Bariatric surgery is one of the most effective means of decreasing the incidence of GDM in obese women.[12-17] A meta-analysis of 15 studies have

Table 26.1: Effects of surgery on occurrence of various complications.

Reduced incidence	*Increased incidence*
GDM	Cesarean section rate
PIH and preeclampsia	Nutritional deficiencies
Lowered gestational weight gain	Mechanical and surgical complications
Fetal macrosomia	IUGR
	Congenital malformation
No effect on BMI	

(GDM: Gestational diabetes mellitus; PIH: Pregnancy induced hypertension; IUGR: Intrauterine growth restriction; BMI: Body mass index)

found that the relative risk reduction of GDM was halved with an overall odds ratio of 0.47.[18] Another meta-analysis showed similar significant reduction but with high heterogeneity.[19] Main reason for decreased GDM is the effective reduction of prepregnancy BMI. Although the interval from surgery to conception does not appear to significantly affect the rate of GDM postoperatively, equivalent rates of GDM have been found during and after the first year after BS,[20] but there are more risk of other fetomaternal complication during the first year post BS.

Effect on Pregnancy Induced Hypertension

There is strong evidence that BS reduces the risk of developing preeclampsia.[9,21,22] Recent meta-analysis has found that surgery cuts the risk of preeclampsia to 50%.[18] Few studies have shown a reduction in the pregnancy induced hypertension (PIH) as high as 75 %.[23]

Risk of Cesarean Section

At the current time, the balance of the evidence indicates that prior BS has no demonstrable effect on the rate of cesarean section (CS). But many studies have reported increase in CS rates which may be because of precious pregnancy, infertility treatment, and high socioeconomic status of these women. It has been found that the risk for CS was slightly increased in second deliveries after BS as opposed to first deliveries which was statistically significant.[24]

Effect on Fetus

Bariatric surgery reduces the risk for macrosomic infants.[12] In general, the neonate born after maternal BS has an increased risk of being small, premature, and requiring admission to the neonatal intensive care unit, but with no significantly increased risk of perinatal mortality.[18] Evidence for specific undernutrition is controversial. Roos et al in their Cohort study[25] found a statistically significant increase in small for gestational age neonates and a decrease in large for gestational age neonates. The reason for small neonates could be maternal malnutrition and microenvironment deficiencies caused by BS. The risk for small neonates appears to be particularly increased after malabsorptive procedures. Subgroup analysis by Galazis et al. showed that women who had undergone LAGB did not have a significant increase in small neonates over women who had not undergone surgery (P = 0.23).[18] This is an important finding, because it suggests restrictive procedures might be preferred in women of childbearing age over malabsorptive procedures. All together, strong evidence indicates a beneficial reduction in large neonates but causes a concerning increase in small neonates born to mothers after BS. Mothers should be counseled regarding the effect of surgery on fetal growth and the risk this effect may result from nutritional deficiencies inherent to malabsorptive surgery.

Risk of Prematurity

There is a 28% increase in preterm births.[18] A Swedish study suggested an increased risk of prematurity in women who had greater decrease in weight during the period from surgery to early pregnancy.[26]

Maternal Anemia and Nutritional Deficiencies

Of all vitamin and mineral deficiencies, there was significant increase in maternal anemia in postoperative women.[18,27,28]

Timing of Conception after Bariatric Surgery

It is highly recommended to delay pregnancy for 12–18 months after surgery, because of a rapid weight loss phase and its specific stressful influence on the organs. Perinatal outcomes and complications of pregnancy were similar for pregnancies conceived early (<12 months after surgery) versus late (>12 or >18 months after surgery).[29] Preterm deliveries occurred with higher frequency in pregnancies conceived within the first year after surgery. No difference has been observed in the incidence of GDM, PIH, CS, birth weight, intrauterine growth restriction (IUGR), or small for gestational age (SGA), between early or late groups.

Antenatal Care

Antenatal care in post-BS needs multidisciplinary approach involving the obstetrician, the bariatric surgeon and the nutritionist. Early consultation is needed to determine baseline nutritional status along with regular checkups. Screening for congenital malformation with triple and quadruple test should be done along with level 2 scan.

Screening for GDM is a challenge for post-BS pregnant women. GDM screening with glucose is not possible because of many reasons:

- There are increased chances of dumping syndrome after ingestion of 75/100 g glucose (abdominal pain, cramping, nausea, diarrhea, flushing, tachycardia, and syncope).[30]
- It has also been suggested that International Association of Diabetes and Pregnancy Study Groups (IADPSG) diagnostic criteria in post RYGB women increased the prevalence of GDM diagnosis without changing the pregnancy outcome. Moreover there are more chances of reactive hypoglycemia in these patients.[31]

Screening in GDM can be done by fasting and postprandial blood sugar levels or continuous blood glucose monitoring for 1 week between 24 gestational weeks and 28 gestational weeks or by HbA1c to avoid this risk of dumping syndrome.[22]

Nutritional Supplementation

Periodic clinical and biochemical monitoring is recommended after malabsorptive surgeries even if patient is tolerating the diet adequately without vomiting and diarrhea so as to detect subclinical nutritional deficiencies. Patients should be tested regularly for complete blood count, glucose, electrolytes, and creatinine every 3 months for the first year after surgeries and albumin, iron, B12, folate, calcium, and vitamin D every 6 months in the first year and then repeated yearly. Restrictive procedure also may require testing if there is poor tolerance to food. In pregnancy these tests can be performed once in each trimester if levels are normal. Persistent deficiencies may require frequent testing and consultation with bariatric surgeon.

There is no standard approach to screening and treatment of deficiencies. The recommendation varies with the type of the procedure performed with a close surveillance after malabsorptive procedures (RYGB). Selective deficiencies are less common after LAGB.

- *Protein supplementation:* It is same and daily 60 g of protein is required.
- *Calcium supplementation:* It is advised to increase the intake of 1,000 mg of calcium during pregnancy to 2,000 mg of calcium citrate with vitamin D (50–150 mcg).The citrate form is preferred as it does not require acidic environment for absorption.[32]
- *Iron supplementation:* Iron deficiency in these patients is caused by achlorhydria or bypass of duodenum and proximal jejunum which are the first and main site of the iron absorption. The important points to remember during supplementation in these patients are:
    - Ferrous form should be supplemented to avoid the need of acidic environment.
    - Recommended 30 mg of daily iron supplementation to be increased to 40–65 mg daily.

  - Regular estimation of serum levels of hemoglobin, iron, ferritin, and transferrin is mandatory so that the dose of iron can be modified accordingly.
- *Vitamin B12 supplementation:* Vitamin B12 deficiency occur due to the absence of acid environment, inadequate secretion of intrinsic factor (IF) and malabsorption. The recommended daily sublingual dose of cobalamin during pregnancy after BS should be increased from 3 mcg to 10 mcg in easily absorbed crystalline form. Intramuscular injections in monthly dose 1,000 mcg can also be used.
- *Folic acid supplementation:* Prenatal supplementation with vitamins containing 4 mg of folic acid prior to and during pregnancy is usually sufficient to maintain adequate serum levels to reduce the risk of neural tube defects.
- *Vitamin A supplementation:* It is reported that this deficiency exists in 10% of patients following gastric bypass. Vitamin A is also needed for normal fetal lung development and maturation. Moreover, vitamin A deficiency also increases susceptibility to respiratory infections and diarrhea. Vitamin A stores in the fetal liver is affected by the maternal vitamin A levels thus plasma retinol levels must be examined periodically and if necessary oral supplement therapy in dose of 5,000 IU/day can be given.
- *Vitamin K supplementation:* Excessive vomiting or fat malabsorption may lead to a higher risk of vitamin K-deficient bleeding disorders of the neonates. Eerdekens et al, reported on five cases with severe intracranial bleeding and skeletal malformations caused by vitamin K deficiency of mothers following BS. However, there are no recommendations about supplementation of the vitamin K.
- *Zinc supplementation:* Recommendations is same as in routine pregnant woman.
- *Iodide supplementation:* There are no recommendations for the pregnant women after bariatric treatment. Due to the threat of malnutrition the daily intake of 250 mcg of iodide is recommended as against 150 mcg in routine pregnancy.

CONCLUSION

BS is becoming a popular alternative to treat obesity and it's related complications. Pregnancy after BS has less risk of developing GDM but requires constant monitoring and supervision through a multidisciplinary team approach.

KEY POINTS

- Bariatric surgery, now known as metabolic surgery is a promising option to cure obesity & associated co-morbidities like DM. Conception should be avoided for 1-1.5 years after BS BS reduces chances of developing GDM,hypertension and macrosomia.

- Pregnancy after BS may lead to an increase in SGA fetus.
- Conventional OGTT should be avoided and diagnosis of GDM should be made by fasting and PP plasma glucose, CGM or by HbA1c.
- Multidisciplinary approach, regular ANC with careful fetal monitoring & nutrient supplements during pregnancy & breastfeeding will give optimum results

REFERENCES

1. Obesity: preventing and managing a global epidemic. Report of a WHO consultation. World Health Organ Tech Rep Ser. 2000;894:i-xii,1-253.
2. World Health Organization. (2012). World Health Statistics 2012. [online] Available from http://www.who.int/gho/publications/world_health_statistics/EN_WHS2012_Full.pdf [Accessed December 2017].
3. Ogden CL, Carroll MD, Fryar CD, et al. Prevalence of obesity among adults and youth: United states, 2011-2014. NCHS Data Brief. 2015;219:1-8.
4. NFHS-4 2015-2016. India Fact Sheet. [online] Available from http://rchiips.org/nfhs/pdf/NFHS4/India.pdf [Accessed December 2017].
5. Canadian Institute for Health Information. (2014). Bariatric surgery in Canada. [online] Available from https://secure.cihi.ca/free_products/Bariatric_Surgery_in_Canada_EN.pdf [Accessed December 2017].
6. Catalano PM. Trying to understand gestational diabetes. Diabet Med. 2014;31: 273-81.
7. Buchwals H, Avidor Y, Braunwald E, et al. Bariatric surgery: a systematic review and meta-analysis. JAMA. 2004;292:1724-37.
8. Adams TD, Gress RE, Smith SC, et al. Long-term mortality after gastric bypass surgery. N Eng J Med. 2007;357:753-61.
9. Sjostrom L, Narbro K, Sjostorm CD, et al. Effects of bariatric surgery on mortality in Swedish obese subjects. N Engl J Med. 2007;357:741-52.
10. Ikramuddin S, Buchwald H. How bariatric and metabolic operations control metabolic syndrome. Br J Surg. 2011;98:1339-41.
11. Leslie DB, Dorman RB, Serrot FJ, et al. Efficacy of the Roux-en-Y gastric bypass compared to medically managed controls in meeting the American Diabetes Association composite end point goals for management of type 2 diabetes mellitus. Obes Surg. 2012;22:367-74.
12. Sebire NJ, Jolly M, Harris JP, et al. Maternal obesity and pregnancy outcome: a study of 287,213 pregnancy in London. Int J Obes Relat Metab Disord. 2001;25:1175-82.
13. Lu GC, Rouse DJ, Dubard M, et al. The effect of the prevalence of maternal obesity on perinatal morbidity. Am J Obstet Gynecol. 2001;185:845-9.
14. Sheiner E, Willis K, Yogev Y. Bariatric surgery: impact on pregnancy outcomes. Curr Diab Rep. 2012;13:19-26.
15. Vrebosch L, Bel S,Vansant G. Maternal and neonatal outcome after laparoscopic adjustable gastric banding: a systematic review. Obes Surg. 2012;22:1568-79.
16. Willis K, Sheiner E. Bariatric surgery and pregnancy: the magical solution? J Perinat Med. 2013;41:133-40.
17. Willis K, Lieberman N, Sheiner E. Pregnancy and neonatal outcome after bariatric surgery. Best Pract Res Clin Obstet Gynaecol. 2014;29:133-44.

18. Galazis N, Docheva N, Simillis C, et al. Maternal and neonatal outcomes in women undergoing bariatric surgery: a systematic review and meta-analysis. Eur J Obstet Gynecol Reprod Biol. 2014;181:45-53.
19. Yi XY, Li QF, Zhang J, et al. A meta-analysis of maternal and fetal outcomes of pregnancy after bariatric surgery. Int J Gynecol Obstet. 2015;130:3-9.
20. Sheiner E, Edri A, Balaban E, et al. Pregnancy outcome of patients who conceive during or after the first year following bariatric surgery. Am J Obstet Gynecol. 2011; 204:50.e1-6.
21. Kominiarek MA. Preparing for and managing a pregnancy after bariatric surgery. Semin Perinatol. 2011;35:356-61.
22. Guelinckx I, Devlieger R, Donceel P, et al. Lifestyle after bariatric surgery: a multicenter, prospective cohort study in pregnant women. Obes Surg. 2012;22: 1456-64.
23. Bennett WL, Gilson MM, Jamshidi R, et al. Impact of bariatric surgery on hypertensive disorders in pregnancy: retrospective analysis of insurance claims data. BMJ. 2010; 340:c1662.
24. Amsalem D, Aricha-Tamir B, LeviI, et al. Obstetric outcomes after restrictive bariatric surgery: what happens after 2 consecutive pregnancies? Surg Obes Relat Dis. 2013; 10:445-9.
25. Roos N, Neovius M, Cnattingius S, et al. Perinatal outcomes after bariatric surgery: nationwide population based matched cohort study. BMJ. 2013;347: f6460.
26. Johansson K, Cnattingius S, Näslund I, et al. Outcomes of pregnancy after bariatric surgery. N Engl J Med. 2015;372:814-24.
27. Shai D, Shoham-Vardi I, Amsalem D, et al. Pregnancy outcome of patients following bariatric surgery as compared with obese women: a population-based study. J Matern Fetal Neonatal Med. 2013;27:1-4.
28. Aricha-Tamir B, Weintraub AY, Levi I, et al. Downsizing pregnancy complications: a study of paired pregnancy outcomes before and after bariatric surgery. Surg Obes Relat Dis. 2012;8:434-9.
29. Martin LF, Finigan KM, Nolan TE. Pregnancy after adjustable gastric banding. Obstet Gynecol. 2000;95(6):927-30.
30. Ukleja A. Dumping syndrome: pathophysiology and treatment: Nutr Clin Pract. 2005; 20:517-25.
31. Freitas C, Araujo C, Rita Caldas, et al. Effect of new criteria of gestational diabetes in women submitted to gastric bypass. Sur Obes Relat Dis. 2014;10:1041-46.
32. Goode LR, Brolin RE, Chowdhary AH, et al. Bone loss and gastric bypass surgery: effects of dietary calcium and vitamin D. Obes Res. 2004;12:40-7.

CHAPTER 27

Fertility Issues with Hyperglycemia

Sonia Malik, Neeti Chhabra

INTRODUCTION

Diabetes mellitus has become a global pandemic. According to WHO statistics, the number of people with diabetes mellitus have risen from 108 million in 1980 to 422 million in 2014.[1] The global prevalence among adults over the age of 18 years has risen from 4.7% in 1980 to 8.5% in 2014.[1] In 2015, an estimated 1.6 million deaths were directly caused by diabetes. Another 2.2 million deaths were attributable to high blood glucose in 2012. WHO projects that diabetes will be the seventh leading cause of death in 2030.[1] The prevalence is rising more rapidly in middle and low income countries. The incidence of type 1 diabetes is rising at a rate of 3% per year. Due to increasing incidence of obesity in children and adolescents, the incidence of type 2 diabetes is also increasing in both underdeveloped and developing nations.[2]

Infertility is defined as the inability to conceive after 1 year of regular unprotected intercourse. The incidence of infertility is on the rise. It nowadays, is not just a problem due to health but due to choices of people's lifestyle. During recent decades, interest of health scientists has turned to investigating the factors that affect fertility, firstly because more and more countries are facing it and secondly because the procreation and upbringing of children is an extremely important life event.

How does Diabetes Lead to Infertility?

Diabetes mellitus is a metabolic disorder. It mainly involves abnormality of carbohydrate metabolism. The disease process is multipronged and has widespread ramifications. It involves vital organs such as eyes, nerves, kidneys, liver, blood vessels, and reproductive tissues as well. Type 1 diabetics are genetically predisposed and it gets activated by the environmental factors. There is an autoimmune response to beta cells of pancreas that produce insulin. Islet cell antibodies are formed to destroy the population of β-cell in the pancreas thereby affecting insulin secretion.[3]

Hyperglycemia and diabetes are implicated as causative and contributory factors in the development of subfertility and infertility in both men and women. Diabetic men have increased incidence of sexual dysfunctions.[2] About 35–75% of these men will experience some form of erectile dysfunction. Others experience reduced libido.[2] Onset of erectile dysfunction follows the onset of the disease, with it occurring earlier in those who have early onset of uncontrolled diabetes type 1. Reduced testicular mitochondrial function is implicated in the pathogenesis. Diabetes type 1 is associated with autoimmune orchitis which leads to impaired spermatogenesis and subfertility. Diabetic men have increased reactive oxidative species (ROS) levels in the semen which results from uncontrolled hyperglycemia. This leads to increased oxidation of lipids, proteins and DNA. Increased mitochondrial and nuclear DNA damage due to increased oxidative stress also adds to the abnormal sperm morphology (<4% normal forms) and increased DNA fragmentation index (> 30%) in these patients.[4]

Reduced testosterone levels in diabetic men occur due to impaired Leydig cell function which in turn causes hypospermatogenesis.[4] Diabetic infertile men may experience retrograde ejaculation which contributes to infertility in them. Men with diabetes have abnormal semen analysis parameters with oligoasthenoteratospermia. These occur in about 50% of subfertile couples. There is low semen pH and volume.[4] Semen levels of interleukin-17 (IL-17) and IL-18 are raised which contribute to the oxidative stress in the testes.[4]

Menstrual irregularities: Women with diabetes experience delayed menarche, oligomenorrhea, secondary amenorrhea, and early menopause.[2] A disturbed hypothalamo pituitary ovarian axis leads to these irregularities. Before the advent of Insulin in the market for treatment of type 1 diabetes, young girls with the disease did not attain menarche. When it did occur, menses usually ceased early. Only 2% of type 1 diabetic women achieved successful pregnancy.[2] According to a study by Strotmeyer,[5] type 1 diabetes was independently associated with oligomenorrhea (> 31 days), menorrhagia (> 7 days of flow or heavy flow). Type 1 diabetic women with low BMI have intracellular starvation due to nutritional restrictions and certain catabolic processes especially before starting insulin. The mechanism of action is very similar to what operates in Anorexia nervosa. This leads to a disruption in the HPO axis and affects the pulsatile release of gonadotropin-releasing hormone (GnRH) and subsequent gonadotropins.[2]

Also, the pituitary gland becomes less sensitive to GnRH from the hypothalamus.[6] The menstrual disturbances in type 1 diabetics are mainly hypothalamic in origin than primary pituitary as it was seen that the response of luteinizing hormone (LH) to exogenous GnRH was different. GnRH secretion from the hypothalamus is also inhibited by increased central dopaminergic activity.[7] It is seen that type 1 diabetics with menstrual abnormalities had lower prolactin levels.[7] Endogenous opium like peptides—endorphins also have an inhibitory effect on GnRH release.[8]

Hyperandrogenism and polycystic ovary syndrome (PCOS)-Type 1 diabetics are also associated with PCOS. Insulin therapy in high doses for the treatment of type 1 diabetes may lead to hyperandrogenism and PCOS. Insulin resistance in type 1 diabetics contributes in the same manner. Risk factors for type 2 diabetes like sedentary lifestyle, obesity, dyslipidemia, and hyperinsulinemia are independent risk factors for infertility.[2] Hyperinsulinemia causes hyperandrogenemia due to increased secretion from the adrenals and ovaries through alteration in the levels of insulin-like growth factor 1 (IGF-1), insulin-like growth factor-binding protein (IGFBP) and sex hormone-binding globulin (SHBG). Polycystic ovary (PCO) women are at increased risk of type 3 diabetes mellitus as was shown by Legro et al.[9].

Obesity: Obesity is an independent risk factor for diabetes. The time to conception increases with increase in the BMI. Obese women have poor egg and embryo quality. Studies have shown increased levels of insulin, triglyceride, lipoprotein receptor, C-reactive protein and free androgen levels in the follicular fluid of obese women. Bariatric surgery has shown improvements in the hormones leading to normalization of menses, fertility, and pregnancy outcomes.[10-13]

Autoimmunity oophoritis occurs as a part of polyglandular autoimmune failure associated with autoantibodies against multiple endocrine organs. Ovarian autoantibodies are present in 67.9% of type 1 diabetics as compared to 4.8% healthy controls. These antibodies affect the ovarian steroid-producing cells and lead to premature ovarian failure.[2]

Sexual dysfunction: Diabetes causes sexual dysfunctions not only in men but also women. Uncontrolled diabetes causes impaired sexual arousal. There is inadequate lubrication leading to dyspareunia, limited sexual desire and sexual activity around the time of ovulation contributing to low fertility.[2]

Genital infections: Uncontrolled diabetics have increased episodes of lower genital infections which may ascend and cause pelvic inflammatory disease (PID). PID is a known cause of tubal blockade and thus infertility. This may lead to dense adhesions in the pelvis with increased risk of trauma to the viscera during egg retrieval. Poor oocyte quality leading to poor embryo quality also results from such florid pelvic infections.

Premature menopause: Type 1 diabetics were almost twice as likely to experience menopause earlier than nondiabetic women. Women who attained early menopause were also those who had early onset of type 1 diabetes.[2] Type 1 diabetics attain menopause about 10 years earlier than nondiabetic sisters and unrelated diabetic controls.[14] The reason for premature menopause in these patients is the cell senescence that occurs due to the catabolic disease process and autoimmunity due to ovarian autoantibodies.[2]

RISK FACTORS COMMON FOR INFERTILITY AND HYPERGLYCEMIA

The following risk factors are common between infertility and hyperglycemia:

- Sedentary lifestyle and obesity

- Chronic oligo- and anovulation, e.g. PCOS, hypothyroidism
- Advancing age more than 40 years
- Metabolic syndrome
- Asian ethnicity with earlier menopause than Caucasians
- History of gestational diabetes mellitus and macrosomia in the previous pregnancy.

Metabolic Syndrome

It is the name given to a group of risk factors that occur together and increase the risk for coronary artery disease, stroke, and type 2 diabetes. Metabolic syndrome is present if there are three or more of the following signs:

1. Blood pressure equal to or higher than 130/85 mm Hg.
2. Fasting blood sugar (glucose) equal to or higher than 100 mg/dL
3. Large waist circumference (length around the waist):
   - *Men*: 40 inches or more
   - *Women*: 35 inches or more
4. Low high-density lipoprotein (HDL) cholesterol:
   - *Men*: Under 40 mg/dL
   - *Women*: Under 50 mg/dL
5. Triglycerides equal to or higher than 150 mg/dL.

The typical weight distribution in such cases is around the middle and upper parts of the body (central obesity). The body may be described as "apple-shaped". The body uses insulin less effectively than normal. Insulin is needed to help control the amount of sugar in the body. As a result, blood sugar and fat levels rise. The prevalence of metabolic syndrome in women with PCOS (mean SD age, 43.0 ± 5.8 years) was 23.8% according to a study by Hudecova et al.[15] Not all PCOS phenotypes have similar metabolic risk. The combination of hyperandrogenemia and oligomenorrhea signifies the most at risk group (level B).[16]

According to American Diabetes Association (ADA) guidelines 2017, risk factors for prediabetes and type 2 diabetes mellitus are:[17]

- HbA1C more than or equal to 5.7% (39 mmol/mol), impaired glucose tolerance (IGT) or impaired fasting glucose (IFG) on previous testing
- First-degree relative with diabetes
- High-risk race/ethnicity (e.g. African American, Latino, Native American, Asian American, Pacific Islander)
- Women who were diagnosed with GDM
- History of cardiovascular disease (CVD)
- Hypertension (≥140/90 mm Hg or on therapy for hypertension)
- High-density lipoprotein cholesterol level less than 35 mg/dL (0.90 mmol/L) and/or a triglyceride level more than 250 mg/dL (2.82 mmol/L)
- Women with PCOS
- Physical inactivity

- Other clinical conditions associated with insulin resistance (e.g. severe obesity, acanthosis nigricans).

American Diabetes Association guidelines for screening for prediabetes and diabetes:[17]

- Screening for prediabetes and diabetes with an informal assessment of risk factors or validated tools should be considered in asymptomatic adults (level B)
- Testing should begin at age 45 years for all people (level B)
- Consider testing for prediabetes and diabetes in asymptomatic adults of any age with BMI more than or equal to 25 kg/m^2 or more than or equal to 23 kg/m^2 (in Asian Americans) who have one or more additional risk factors for diabetes (level B)
- If tests are normal, repeat at a minimum of 3-year intervals (level C)
- Fasting plasma glucose (FPG), 2-h PG after 75-g OGTT (oral glucose tolerance test), and A_{1C}, are equally appropriate for prediabetes and diabetes testing (level B)
- In patients with prediabetes and diabetes, identify and if appropriate, treat other CVD risk factors (level B)
- Consider prediabetes and diabetes testing in overweight/obese children and adolescents with 2 or more additional diabetes risk factors (level E).

According to American Diabetes Association, the criteria for testing for type 2 diabetes mellitus in children and adolescents are as follows:[17]

- Overweight plus any two:
  - Family history of type 2 diabetes in first or second degree relative
  - Race/ethnicity
  - Signs of insulin resistance or conditions associated with insulin resistance
  - Maternal history of diabetes or GDM.
- Age of initiation 10 years or at onset of puberty
- Frequency of testing : every 3 years
- Test with FPG, OGTT, or HbA1C.

DIAGNOSIS

According to ADA standards of medical care in diabetes, the following criteria are used for the diagnosis:[17]

Prediabetes

FPG 100–125 mg/dL (5.6–6.9 mmol/L): IFG
OR
2-hours plasma glucose 140–199 mg/dL (7.8–11.0 mmol/L): IGT
OR
A1C 5.7–6.4%.

Diagnosis of Diabetes

Fasting plasma glucose ≥126 mg/dL (7.0 mmol/L)
OR
2-hours plasma glucose ≥200 mg/dL (11.1 mmol/L) during an OGTT
OR
HbA1C ≥6.5%
OR
Classic diabetes symptoms + random plasma glucose ≥200 mg/dL (11.1 mmol/L).

MANAGEMENT

The management of IGT and diabetes involves a multidisciplinary team approach. The presence of the disease process has widespread ramifications with impact on almost all the systems of the body. With the ever increasing levels of stress in today's society, the impact of the disease process is many folds. Therefore screening and diagnosis at the earliest is important and once diagnosed early, prompt and effective management can reverse the damages done.

The management of hyperglycemia for improving fertility involves:
- Lifestyle management
- Drugs.

Lifestyle Management

Physical Activity

Increasing physical activity is the first-line therapy for the treatment of PCOS, metabolic syndrome and hyperglycemia. As all these are inter-related, exercise does improve the disease process and prevents disease progression. The benefits of physical activity (at least 150 min/week) in improving metabolic status and reducing the incidence of diabetes in high-risk groups of general population have been reported. In adults and adolescents with PCOS, daily strict physical activity sessions for at least 30 min/day or 150 min/week are recommended (Grade A, EL 4).[18]

Diet Control

In women at risk for hyperglycemia, weight loss through diet control has been shown to improve pregnancy rates, normalize hyperandrogenemia, and improve insulin sensitivity, menstrual functions, and hirsutism. For the management of obesity in adults (BMI >23 kg/m) and adolescents (BMI >97.5 percentile for age) with PCOS, it is recommended to follow lifestyle modifications in combination with healthy, balanced diet consisting of regular, calorie-restricted meals (Grade B, EL 4).[18] In adult and adolescent women with PCOS, it is recommended to routinely screen for BMI and waist circumference as an index for increasing adiposity and development of hyperandrogenism (Grade A, EL 3).[18] It is recommended to follow calorie-restricted diet (low carbohydrate and fat, high protein) in consultation with dietician and lifestyle modification as first-line therapy for at least 6 months, then add metformin as second-line therapy (Grade B, EL 4).[18]

Pharmacotherapy

- Insulin
- Oral hypoglycemic agents.

ORAL HYPOGLYCEMIC AGENTS: METFORMIN AND INOSITOLS AND THEIR APPLICATION IN INFERTILITY

Metformin

Metformin was first introduced in 1957 with phenformin but got popularized only in 1970s after phenformin was withdrawn from market because of high incidence of lactic acidosis. Metformin is commonly used in the treatment of insulin resistance manifesting as type 2 diabetes or PCOS. With an increasing number of these patient conceiving, its use in and around pregnancy has increased.

Pharmacodynamics and Pharmacokinetics

Metformin is a dimethyl biguanide—only biguanide that is used now days.

1. It increases tyrosine kinase activity
2. Activates adenosine monophosphate (AMP)-activated protein kinases involved in fatty acid and glucose metabolism
3. Increases IP_3 (inositol-3,4,5-triphosphate)
4. Increases intracellular free calcium
5. Increased phosphorylation of insulin receptor substitutes.

Insulin stimulated flux of glucose into cells depends on IP_3—increasing activity and cycling of GLUT4 glucose transporting protein. Metformin augments insulin dependent (GLUT4) and insulin independent (GLUT4 and GLUT3) cellular uptake of glucose.

Pharmacokinetics[19]

- *Bioavailability*: 50–60 percent; absorbed mainly from small intestine; estimated absorption half-life, 0.9–.6 hours.
- *Plasma concentration*: Maximal, 1 to 2 µg/mL (1–2 hours after the oral dose of 500–1,000 mg; negligible binding to phase protein)
- *Plasma half-life*: 1.5–4.9 hours

- *Metabolism*: Not measurably metabolized
- *Elimination*: About 90% is eliminated in urine in 12 hours
- *Tissue distribution*: Distributed in most tissues at concentration similar to those in peripheral plasma, higher concentration in liver and kidney.

Mechanism of Action[20]

It has antihyperglycemic effect by following mechanisms:

- Increased peripheral cellular glucose uptake
- Reduced hepatic gluconeogenesis—contributing to postabsorptive and postprandial plasma glucose lowering effect
- Reduced absorption of glucose
- Reduces basal hepatic glucose output in patients with type 2 diabetes mellitus, providing an important mechanism through which the drug lowers fasting plasma glucose concentration.

Unlike sulfonylureas, hypoglycemia is not an adverse side effect of biguanide because they do not enhance endogenous insulin production. Langer et al. (2000) noted that they do not stimulate β-pancreatic cells to produce insulin. No neonatal hyperinsulinemia was seen in his study when used in pregnant diabetics.

Actions of Metformin in Polycystic Ovary Syndrome

- Reduces hyperinsulinemia
- Decrease in intraovarian androgens
- Reduction in estradiol levels
- Favors orderly follicular growth in response to exogenous gonadotropins
- Decrease in testosterone, free testosterone, dehydroepiandrosterone sulfate (DHEAS), androstenedione luteinizing hormone (LH)
- Normalization of LH: Follicle-stimulating hormone (FSH) ratio
- Increase in SHBG.

Indications for Metformin Use

1. Polycystic ovary syndrome patients with increased androgens
2. Documented ovulation induction failure after clomiphene with BMI more than 25. According to SOGC guidelines 2010,[21] metformin can be added to clomiphene citrate for ovulation induction in women who are older and have visceral obesity.
3. Documented insulin resistance by blood sugar and serum insulin values. According to Thessaloniki ESHRE/ASRM-Sponsored PCOS Consensus Workshop Group[22] there is no clear role for insulin sensitizing and insulin lowering drug in the management of PCOS, and should be restricted to those patients with glucose intolerance or type 2 diabetes rather than those with just insulin resistance.

According to the consensus on women's health aspects of polycystic ovarian syndrome: the Amsterdam ESHRE/ASRM sponsored 3rd polycystic ovary (PCO) consensus workshop group,[23] there is no evidence for improved live-birth rate or decreased pregnancy complications with the use of metformin either before conception or during pregnancy (level A evidence).

According to the polycystic ovary syndrome—evidence-based guidelines, Australia (2011):[24]

Metformin is a category B drug. It is indicated as:

- With clomiphene citrate in CC resistant PCOS (level A)
- With clomiphene citrate in PCOS, BMI more than 30 kg/m^2 (level A)
- Could be used alone to improve ovulation and pregnancy rates in PCOS, BMI less than 30 kg/m^2 (level B).

Cochrane review on the use of insulin-sensitizing drugs [metformin, rosiglitazone, pioglitazone, D-chiro-inositol (DCI)] for women with polycystic ovary syndrome, oligoamenorrhea and subfertility.[25]

Forty-four trials (3,992 women) were included for analysis, 38 of them using metformin and involving 3,495 women. There was no evidence that metformin improved live-birth rates, whether it was used alone [pooled odds ratio (OR) 1.80, 95% confidence interval (CI) 0.52–6.16, 3 trials, 115 women] or in combination with clomiphene (pooled OR 1.16, 95% CI 0.85–1.56, 7 trials, 907 women). However, clinical pregnancy rates were improved for metformin versus placebo (pooled OR 2.31, 95% CI 1.52–3.51, 8 trials, 707 women) and for metformin and clomiphene versus clomiphene alone (pooled OR 1.51, 95% CI 1.17–1.96, 11 trials, 1208 women). In the studies that compared metformin and clomiphene alone, there was evidence of an improved live-birth rate (pooled OR 0.3, 95% CI 0.17–0.52, 2 trials, 500 women) and clinical pregnancy rate (pooled OR 0.34, 95% CI 0.21–0.55, 2 trials, 500 women) in the group of obese women who took clomiphene. Metformin was also associated with a significantly higher incidence of gastrointestinal disturbances than placebo (pooled OR 4.27, 95% CI 2.4–7.59, 5 trials, 318 women) but no serious adverse effects were reported.

Cochrane review on the use of metformin during ovulation induction with gonadotropins followed by timed intercourse or intrauterine insemination for subfertility associated with polycystic ovary syndrome.[26]

Five randomized controlled trials (RCTs) (with 264 women) comparing gonadotropins plus metformin versus gonadotropins alone were included. The gonadotropin used was recombinant FSH in four studies and highly purified FSH in one study. The results were as follows:

Metformin plus FSH was associated with a higher cumulative live birth rate when compared with FSH (OR 2.31, 95% CI 1.23–4.34; two RCTs, n = 180; I2 = 0%; low-quality evidence). This suggests that if the chance of live birth after FSH is assumed to be 27%, then the chance after addition of metformin would be between 32% and 60%. Also metformin use was associated with a higher ongoing pregnancy rate (OR 2.46, 95% CI 1.36–4.46; four RCTs, n = 232; I2 = 0%; low-quality evidence) and a higher clinical pregnancy rate (OR 2.51, 95% CI 1.46–4.31; five RCTs, n = 264; I2 = 0%; low-quality evidence). There was no evidence of a difference in multiple pregnancy rates between metformin plus FSH and FSH (OR 0.55, 95% CI 0.15–1.95; four RCTs, n = 232; I2 = 0%; low-quality evidence) and no evidence of a difference in rates of miscarriage or OHSS.

Cochrane review on the use of metformin treatment before and during IVF or ICSI in women with polycystic ovary syndrome.[27]

Nine randomized controlled trials involving a total of 816 women with PCOS. When metformin was compared with placebo there was no clear evidence of a difference between the groups in live-birth rates (OR 1.39, 95% CI 0.81–2.40, five RCTs, 551 women, I2 = 52%, low-quality evidence). It suggests that for a woman with a 32% chance of achieving a live birth using placebo, the corresponding chance using metformin treatment would be between 28% and 53%. When metformin was compared with placebo or no treatment, clinical pregnancy rates were higher in the metformin group (OR 1.52; 95% CI 1.07–2.15; eight RCTs, 775 women, I2 = 18%, moderate-quality evidence). This suggests that for a woman with a 31% chance of achieving a clinical pregnancy using placebo or no treatment, the corresponding chance using metformin treatment would be between 32% and 49%.

The risk of ovarian hyperstimulation syndrome was lower in the metformin group (OR 0.29; 95% CI 0.18–0.49, eight RCTs, 798 women, I2 = 11%, moderate-quality evidence). This suggests that for a woman with a 27% risk of having OHSS without metformin the corresponding chance using metformin treatment would be between 6% and 15%. Side effects (mostly gastrointestinal) were more common in the metformin group (OR 4.49, 95% CI 1.88–10.72, for RCTs, 431women, I2 = 57%, low-quality evidence).

Effect of metformin on raised serum anti-Müllerian hormone (AMH) levels in women with PCOS has been studied and an article by the same authors is in press.[28] Insulin sensitizers like metformin reduce serum AMH levels in anovulatory PCO women and convert their cycles into ovulatory. There is a reduction in hyperandrogenism and acne scores also. This improves the chances of spontaneous conception and pregnancy results post-ART (assisted reproductive technology).

Contraindications for Metformin Use

- *Renal impairment*: Plasma creatinine values more than or equal to 1.5 mg/dL
- Cardiac or respiratory insufficiency that in likely to cause central hypoxia or reduced peripheral perfusion
- History of lactic acidosis
- Severe infection that could lead to decreased tissue perfusion

- Liver disease including alcoholic liver disease, as demonstrated by abnormal liver function tests
- Alcohol abuse with binge drinking sufficient to cause acute hepatic toxicity
- Use of intravenous radiographic contrast agents (reported occurrence of lactic acidosis after its use).

Initiating and Monitoring Therapy with Metformin

Metformin has potential advantage of targeting insulin resistance, thus reducing plasma insulin levels. Metformin also reduces adipose tissue mass. The risk of hypoglycemia is much less with metformin as compared to other hypoglycemic agents (insulin).

Metformin should be taken with meals, (to decrease/prevent gastrointestinal side effects). Starting dose of 500 mg twice a day, which can slowly be increased up to 2 gm/day. Patients starting metformin therapy should have baseline liver function test and renal function test. Also, patients should be advised that they may have minor gastrointestinal side effects. These include diarrhea, abdominal discomfort, anorexia, nausea, and rarely, a metallic taste in mouth.

The symptoms are dose related and reduce if the dose is decreased.

Safety of Metformin in the Peri- and Postconception Period

Since metformin crosses the placenta, its safety in pregnancy for the mother and fetus needs to be ascertained. Studies done in South Africa where it has been used since late 1970s suggest its benefits in women with type 2 diabetes and GDM. The perinatal mortality was higher than the general obstetric population but lower than the untreated and similar to those who used insulin.[29-32] Two meta-analysis of observational studies,[33,34] one of women using metformin and or sulfonyl ureas and one of women using metformin alone during the first trimester did not show an increase in the congenital malformation or neonatal deaths. In another study done in women with type 2 diabetes, the maternal and fetal outcomes were similar in the metformin and insulin groups. In the Metformin in Gestational Diabetes Trial (MiG Trial), 751 women were randomized to receive either metformin or insulin, the women in the metformin group had less weight gain as compared to the insulin group.[35] Also, a number of studies regarding the use of metformin in PCOS in the peri- and immediate postconception period have suggested its safety in the same.[36,37] The Metformin in Obese Nondiabetic Pregnant Women (MOP) trial is a multicentered, randomized trial of 2,178 obese pregnant women randomized to receive either metformin or placebo with a primary outcome of birth-weight centile. It would examine whether metformin would play a role in obese nondiabetic pregnant patients. The metformin in women with type 2 diabetes in pregnancy (MiTy) trial[38] is ongoing with randomization of 500 women with type 2 diabetes in pregnancy to receive either metformin or placebo in addition to their usual insulin. They intend to study the composite fetal outcome.

It has been postulated that the major determinant of the body fat distribution is the insulin resistance. Normally the body fat gets distributed in the adipose tissue in the subcutaneous areas of the body. As the fat stores increase, so does the insulin resistance and this limits the fat storage in the subcutaneous areas. Therefore, the triglycerides are taken up into the visceral stores and other ectopic sites like liver.[39] Infants exposed to diabetes in utero have increased incidence of childhood obesity and diabetes. It has been suggested by Rowan et al.[40] that metformin helps in a healthier fat distribution in these infants. However, it has to be noted that the earliest effects of diabetes in pregnancy on childhood obesity do not manifest until 6–9 years of age. Hence long-term follow-ups are needed.

Inositols in Polycystic Ovary Syndrome

In 1850 Johannes Scherer isolated inositol from muscle cells and it was formally included in the sugar family. This inositol has been characterized chemically as hexahydroxycyclohexane and has nine stereoisomers. One of these, myo-inositol (myo-ins) is the most common in all biological systems and both myo-ins and DCI are important. They are found in cereals, nuts, fruits, and in human cells.

Mechanism of Action[41]

The inositols are important in glucose homeostasis and serve as second messengers in signal transduction cascade of insulin. Once MYO enters the cell, it is immediately converted to phosphatidyl-myo-inositol, precursor of the IP_3 in the cell membranes. IP_3 acts as intracellular second messenger for insulin as well as for FSH and TSH. Not only MYO but also DCI, is involved in the intracellular transmission of insulin metabolic signal through another mechanism. Both MYO and DCI have the same chemical structure but differ in position of a hydroxyl group. In vivo, DCI is synthesized from MYO by the activity of an epimerase which is insulin stimulated and NAD dependent. Myo-inositol increases glucose cellular uptake and DCI is involved in glycogen synthesis. In fact, cells responsible for glycogen storage (such as liver, muscles, and fat cells) contain high levels of DCI, whereas brain and heart cells contain high concentration of myo-ins, since they require high consumption of glucose.

Polycystic Ovary and Inositol Deficiency[41]

In PCO women, the metabolism of inositols is dysregulated. The insulin resistance and compensatory hyperinsulinemia due to dysregulation of inositol metabolism may actually be the major underlying cause of the disorder. It was shown that an increased activity of epimerase in theca cells of ovaries of PCOS women is associated with a reduction in the intraovarian ratio of myo-ins to DCI. This causes oligoovulation and poor oocyte quality. Thus, myo-ins and DCI supplementation in a physiological ratio (40:1) is important to restore normal ovarian function. This is called the DCI paradox according to which myo-ins rather than DCI improved oocyte quality in intracytoplasmic sperm injection cycles. There is a synergistic action of myo-ins and DCI in overweight PCOS women as myo-ins improves the ovulatory function and DCI rapidly reduces the peripheral hyperinsulinemia.

It has also been seen that hormonal parameters improved significantly in all PCOS patients treated with myo-ins. There is a reduction in the body weight and circulating leptin levels decreased with an increase in HDL concentrations. This may prove to be cardioprotective in PCOS women. The dose of gonadotropins and the duration of stimulation is greatly reduced when myo-ins was given to PCOS during IVF cycles. Myo-inositols also improve the pregnancy rate in PCOS women. Supplementation also reduces the number of germinal vesicle and immature oocytes with an increase in the mature oocyte numbers.

KEY POINTS

- Diabetes Mellitus is a global pandemic with widespread health ramifications including infertility.
- Uncontrolled diabetes affects both male and female Fertility.
- Diabetic males with uncontrolled blood sugar levels have sexual dysfunction, impaired spermatogenesis ,increased sperm DNA damage and abnormal semen parameters.
- Diabetic females with uncontrolled blood sugars have menstrual irregularities ,sexual dysfunction and increased propensity towards genital infections.
- Uncontrolled diabetes is associated with PCOS and hyperandrogenism, obesity and premature menopause.
- Patients at risk for Pre Diabetes and Type II Diabetes need to be screened according to the ADA guidelines 2017.
- Management of Diabetes involves a holistic approach which includes lifestyle management and pharmacotherapy.
- The two most important drugs implicated in the treatment of PCOS are Metformin and Inositols.
- Metformin and inositols improve oocyte quality in infertile PCO patients and convert anovulatory cycles to ovulatory.

REFERENCES

1. Mathers CD, Loncar D. Projections of global mortality and burden of disease from 2002 to 2030. PLoS Med. 2006;11:e442.
2. Livshits A, Seidman DS. Fertility issues in women with diabetes. Womens Health (Lond). 2009;5:701-7.
3. Delfino M, Imbrogno N, Elia J, et al. Prevalence of diabetes mellitus in male partners of infertile couples. Minerva Urol Nefrol. 2007;59:131-5.
4. Basmatzou T, Hatziveis K. Diabetes Mellitus and Influences on Human Fertility. Int J Caring Sci. 2016;9:371.
5. Strotmeyer ES, Steenkiste AR, Foley TP Jr, et al. Menstrual cycle differences between women with type 1 diabetes and women without diabetes. Diabetes Care. 2003;26:1016-21.
6. Johnson LM, Sidman RL. A reproductive endocrine profile in the diabetes (db) mutant mouse. Biol Reprod. 1979;20:552-9.
7. Djursing H, Hagen C, Nyholm HC, et al. Gonadotropin responses to gonadotropin-releasing hormone and prolactin responses to thyrotropin-releasing hormone and metoclopramide in women with amenorrhea and insulin-treated diabetes mellitus. J Clin Endocrinol Metab. 1983;56:1016-21.
8. Arrais RF, Dib SA. The hypothalamus-pituitary-ovary axis and type 1 diabetes mellitus: a mini review. Hum Reprod. 2006;2:327-37.
9. Legro RS, Kunselman AR, Dodson WC, et al. Prevalence and predictors of risk for type 2 diabetes mellitus and impaired glucose tolerance in polycystic ovary syndrome: a prospective, controlled study in 254 affected women. J Clin Endocrinol Metab. 1999;84:165-9.
10. van der Steeg JW, Steures P, Eijkemans MJ, et al. Obesity affects spontaneous pregnancy chances in subfertile, ovulatory women. Hum Reprod. 2007;23:324-8.
11. Jensen TK, Scheike T, Keiding N, et al. Fecundability in relation to body mass and menstrual cycle patterns. Epidemiology. 1999;10:422-8.
12. Metwally M, Cutting R, Tipton A, et al. Effect of increased body mass index on oocyte and embryo quality in IVF patients. Reprod Biomed Online. 2007;15:532-8.
13. Robker RL, Akison LK, Bennett BD, et al. Obese women exhibit differences in ovarian metabolites, hormones, and gene expression compared with moderate weight women. J Clin Endocrinol Metab. 2009;94:1533-40.
14. Dorman JS, Steenkiste AR, Foley TP, et al. Menopause in type 1 diabetic women: is it premature? Diabetes. 2001;50:1857-62.
15. Hudecova M, Holte J, Olovsson M, et al. Prevalence of the metabolic syndrome in women with a previous diagnosis of polycystic ovary syndrome: long-term follow-up. Fertil Steril. 2011;96:1271-4.
16. Fauser B, Tarlatzis BC, Rebar RW, et al. Consensus on women's health aspects of polycystic ovary syndrome (PCOS): the Amsterdam ESHRE/ASRM-Sponsored 3rd PCOS Consensus Workshop Group. Fertil Steril. 2012;97(1): 28-38.e25.
17. American Diabetic Association. Standards of Medical care in Diabetes. Virginia: American Diabetic Association; 2017.
18. Malik S. Management of Polycystic Ovary Syndrome:Consensus Evidence-based Good Clinical Practice Recommendations. New Delhi: Indian Fertility Society; 2015.
19. Alastair JJ, Wood MD, Metformin. N Engl J Med. 2000;334:574-9.
20. Wiernsperger NF, Bailey CJ. The antihyperglycaemic effect of metformin: therapeutic and cellular mechanisms. Drugs. 1999;58:31-9; discussion 75-82.
21. SOGC. (2010). Clinical Practice guidelines. [online] Available from https://sogc.org/clinical-practice-guidelines.html. [Accessed December, 2017].

22. Thessaloniki ESHRE/ASRM-Sponsored PCOS Consensus Workshop Group. Consensus on infertility treatment related to polycystic ovary syndrome. Hum Reprod. 2008;23:462-77.
23. Fauser BC, Tarlatzis BC, Rebar RW, et al. Consensus on women's health aspects of polycystic ovary syndrome (PCOS): the Amsterdam ESHRE/ASRM-Sponsored 3rd PCOS Consensus Workshop Group. Fertil Steril. 2012;97:28-38. e25.
24. CREPCOS. (2011). PCOS—Evidence based guidelines. [online] Available from http://pcos-cre.edu.au/evidence-based-guideline/. [Accessed December, 2017].
25. Tang T, Lord JM, Norman RJ, et al. Insulin-sensitising drugs (metformin, rosiglitazone, pioglitazone, D-chiro-inositol) for women with polycystic ovary syndrome, oligo amenorrhoea and subfertility. Cochrane Database Syst Rev. 2012;5:CD003053.
26. Bordewijk EM, Nahuis M, Costello MF, et al. Metformin during ovulation induction with gonadotrophins followed by timed intercourse or intrauterine insemination for subfertility associated with polycystic ovary syndrome. Cochrane Database Syst Rev. 2017;1:CD009090.
27. Tso LO, Costello MF, Albuquerque LE, et al. Metformin treatment before and during IVF or ICSI in women with polycystic ovary syndrome. Cochrane Database Syst Rev. 2009;2:CD006105.
28. Chhabra N, Malik S. Effect of Insulin sensitizers on raised serum AMH levels in infertile women with PCOS (in press).
29. Coetzee EJ, Jackson WP. Metformin in management of pregnant insulin-independent diabetics. Diabetologia. 1979;16:241-5.
30. Coetzee EJ, Jackson WP. Pregnancy in established non-insulin-dependent diabetics. A five-and-a-half year study at Groote Schuur Hospital. S Afr Med J. 1980;58:795-802.
31. Coetzee EJ, Jackson WP. Oral hypoglycaemics in the first trimester and fetal outcome. S Afr Med J. 1984;65:635-7.
32. Coetzee EJ, Jackson WP. The management of non-insulin-dependent diabetes during pregnancy. Diabetes Res Clin Pract. 1985-1986;1:281-7.
33. Gutzin SJ, Kozer E, Magee LA, et al. The safety of oral hypoglycemic agents in the first trimester of pregnancy: a meta-analysis. Can J Clin Pharmacol. 2003;10:179-83.
34. Gilbert C, Valois M, Koren G. Pregnancy outcome after first-trimester exposure to metformin: a meta-analysis. Fertil Steril. 2006;86:658-63.
35. Rowan JA, Hague WM, Gao W, et al. Metformin versus insulin for the treatment of gestational diabetes. N Engl J Med. 2008;358:2003-15.
36. Tang T, Lord JM, Normal RJ, et al. Insulin-sensitising drugs (metformin, rosiglitazone, pioglitazone, D-chiro-inositol) for women with polycystic ovary syndrome, oligo amenorrhoea and subfertility. Cochrane Database Syst Rev. 2010;4:CD003053.
37. Palomba S, Falbo A, Orio F Jr, et al. Effect of preconceptional metformin on abortion risk in polycystic ovary syndrome: a systematic review and meta-analysis of randomized controlled trials. Fertil Steril. 2009;92:1646-58.
38. US National Library of Medicine. Metformin in Women with Type 2 Diabetes in Pregnancy Trial (MiTy). [online] Available from https://clinicaltrials.gov/ct2/show/NCT01353391 [Accessed December, 2017].
39. Ali AT, Ferris WF, Naran NH, et al. Insulin resistance in the control of body fat distribution: a new hypothesis. Horm Metab Res. 2011;43:77-80.
40. Rowan JA, Rush EC, Obolonkin V, et al. Metformin in Gestational diabetes: The Offspring Follow-Up (MiG TOFU): body composition at 2 years of age. Diabetes Care. 2011;34:2279-84.
41. Unfer V, Nestler JE, Kamenov JA, et al. Effects of Inositol(s) in Women with PCOS: A Systematic Review of Randomized Controlled Trials. Int J Endocrinol. 2016(2016):1849162.

Index

Page numbers followed by *b* refer to box, *f* refer to figure, *fc* refer to flowchart, and *t* refer to table.

C

D

E

F

U

V

W

Z